THE DEVELOPMENT OF VISION

Studies in Developmental Paediatrics

Series Editor Dr Margaret Pollak

Volume 3

THE DEVELOPMENT OF VISION

P. A. Gardiner

Consultant Emeritus in Ophthalmology,
Guy's Hospital, London

MTP PRESS LIMITED International Medical Publishers

Published by
MTP Press Limited
Falcon House
Lancaster, England

Softocve reprint of the hardcover 1st edition 1982
First Published 1982

British Library Cataloguing in Publication Data

Gardiner, P. A.
The development of vision.–(Studies in developmental paediatrics; v.3)
1. Vision
I. Title II. Series
612′.84 QP475

ISBN-13: 978-94-011-7703-0 e-ISBN-13: 978-94-011-7701-6
DOI: 10.1007/978-94-011-7701-6

Printed by Robert MacLehose & Co. Ltd.
Foulis Works, Renfrew

DEDICATION

To Dr Mary Sheridan whose pioneering work laid the solid foundations for the study of so many aspects of child development.

Studies in Developmental Paediatrics

Other books in the series include:

Development of Hearing – Sybil Yeates

Language Development and Assessment – Joan Reynell

Neuromuscular Development – P. Robson

Social Development – Ruth Blunden

Adaptive Development – Margaret Pollak

CONTENTS

SERIES EDITOR'S NOTE

For too long have developmental paediatricians been in the dark as to the correct procedures for – and often the interpretation of – testing the visual competence of babies and young children. Even more have they been unsure how to proceed when a suspected abnormality has been found.

Having been exhorted by the initiated to refer squints 'early' how many of us have been told 'we have to wait until Johnny is older'?

Too often, also, the developmental paediatrician has the skills with which to gain the co-operation of the child but lacks the expertise to test the visual apparatus – whilst for the ophthalmologist the situation is reversed. There is, thus, an obvious need for close co-operation between these two disciplines and it is to be hoped that this will increasingly take place in the future.

This book is based upon the long experience of one of our most gifted paediatric ophthalmologists. Mr Gardiner is a pioneer in his field and has devoted a lifetime to this work. He also had the inestimable advantage of working closely with Mary Sheridan for many years.

He explains, with devastating lucidity, the basic development of vision in the young, the underlying principles of testing and their practical application in the clinical situation, and gives us a vision of how an ideal service for children could look.

This cannot help but be a most useful book – partly because

it contains information which is difficult to obtain elsewhere, and partly because Mr Gardiner has a wealth of clinical experience on which to draw.

I hope it will be widely read amongst all who are concerned with developmental paediatrics and child care.

Margaret Pollak
Consultant Paediatrician to the Sir Wilfrid Sheldon Assessment Centre
Senior Lecturer in Developmental, Social and Educational Paediatrics
King's College Hospital
London SE5

PREFACE

This book is intended to be an aid to all who are concerned with assessing vision and handling day-to-day problems during the growth of infants and children. It is directed mainly to community doctors, health visitors, school nurses, general practitioners, paediatricians and teachers. Members of all these groups have expressed to the author their ignorance and indeed fear of visual problems resulting either in nonchalance or over-anxiety based on the traditional misinformation which most of us have about our eyesight. It is particularly important that nurses and teachers should be able to identify and scale the severity or otherwise of any visual problem.

The book is not primarily one of theory nor does it make any pretence of being weighty or encyclopaedic. It is hoped that it will be of use in conjunction with training courses. Those who wish to go deeper will be helped by the references to further reading. It is inevitable that technical jargon should creep in, but this has been resisted where possible and a glossary has been provided in the hope that anyone interested in children's eyesight will find the book readable.

May 1981

P. A. Gardiner
Guy's Hospital

ACKNOWLEDGEMENTS

I would like to record my thanks to the band of illustrators.
Colin Clements of Guy's Hospital for Figures 6, 13 and 19
Mrs Oliver for the line drawings (Figures 1, 2(b), 3, 4, 5, 7(b), 8, 15 and 16)
Peter Fowler of the John Aird School for the Partially Sighted for Figures 22, 23 and 25
and Messrs. C. Davis Keeler for Figures 12 and 21

There would have been no real chance of this book appearing without all the assistance I have had from my office manager, Mrs Browning, who has kept chaos at bay, typed and retyped impeccably and never failed to supply cake and coffee in the right quantities at the right time.

Chapter 1

INTRODUCTION

> Those first affections
> Those shadowy recollections
> Which, be they what they may,
> Are yet the fountain light of all our day
> Are yet a master light of all our seeing.
>
> Wordsworth

Developmental ophthalmology has only recently been considered worthy of clinical attention. This has come about for many reasons, springing on the one hand from the realization by ophthalmologists that curative procedures in later childhood often were inadequate and too late; and on the other hand from the curiosity and bewilderment of paediatricians anxious to measure and explain retardation of any kind which they believed might have a visual component. The referral of such a child to an ophthalmologist by tradition produced a report often worded in obscure polysyllables, or very simply that no abnormality was to be seen in the ocular tissues nor in the eye movements. The presence of abnormalities would be reported, but their significance might be ignored. As an example, nystagmus in infants would be classified skilfully by the pattern of the abnormal movement, but its possible course and its influence on vision might be left to the paediatrician's imagination. A report that a child had no binocular vision and that the visual acuity was less than 6/60 in one eye might well convince a paediatrician using common sense, especially if he took note of all the treatment prescribed on both counts, that his patient was suffering a severe visual handicap. He might wrongly attribute any aspect of delayed development which might be present to the inferred handicap. This chasm between what the paediatrician wants to know and what is supplied will, it is hoped, be bridged to some extent by this book.

I did not intend to write a textbook of paediatric ophthalmology; neither diseases nor their treatment will be so described, though the significance of such conditions as squints and abnormalities of refraction for the development of acuity and visual behaviour must be considered and the rationale of their treatment explained.

THE VISUAL PROCESS

Vision should provide accurate information so that the organism can react to its environment with versatility. This may be applied to protection, nutrition, to reproduction or, in the higher animals and in particular man, to enable the translation of the external world into concepts and to promote action. Judgement as to what is accurate or inaccurate may be achieved with the other senses; e.g. whether a form is round or flat by touch, whether a granule is sand or pepper by taste, and whether the person in contemporary dress is male or female by the sound of the voice. Dreams and drugs illustrate that the visual process in humans is largely a cerebral activity and that things seen in these conditions do not depend on the eye. When vision is not initiated or controlled by the eye what is seen is of a different and often fantastic nature, however detailed. The eye may therefore be a control of the mind as well as a stimulator and limits what would otherwise be chaos by imposing order on visual impressions. This ordering of visual stimuli depends on intact visual apparatus and on the construction of visual concepts from experience. It is tempting to obtain some insight into the process by talking to children totally blind from birth; but this can be misleading, since they are so used to hearing words with visual meaning that by the time they can convey information the superstructure of customary language covers up their essential ignorance of the nature of sight.

Congenital blindness has been described as similar to what a normal person sees behind them. It is a state not only of ignorance of what is going on visually, but of detachment and disinterest virtually impossible to describe because it is visually non-existent. This idea is supported by the request of a congenitally blind child of 6 years to his ophthalmologist for some sight. He was perfectly satisfied with the answer that there was none available. Sight was something he did not possess and others did – rather like a car or a washing machine – and was only missed in these terms. There is therefore no common content in the meaning of the word when we are discussing sight with the congenitally blind. There is more when we discuss vision which has been lost in victims of disease or accident who have to discard reflexes dependent on vision and for that reason have to rebuild and translate what they can into their visual memory by input from their other senses.

Another aspect of the governing capacity of the eye is shown by the experience of those who in adult life gain vision by surgery, having had little or none before. These people are often disorientated and confused by the flood of new sensation and have the greatest difficulty in making use of their new gift, for which their long experience has provided no suitable context. Their preconceived ideas bear no relationship to the experience of vision and its consequences. These considerations point out the essential relation between the eye and the brain and their interdependence, and also that there is a learning and adaptive mechanism of great significance in the visual process and its interpretation. This is of the greatest importance in considering visual development and if it is ignored the judgements we make as doctors acting solely on our own fully developed experience may be wide of the mark.

Though it needs little thought to see that we all have essentially individual sensory experiences an appropriate illustration is given by considering the ever-changing relationship of the growing child to his environment. The visual opportunities of a tall man are quite different from those of a short one. In the eyes of a man of 195 cm (78 in) tall virtually every other human being is beneath him, whereas to those of few inches the world is populated by superior beings. Therefore the angle of vision also is different between individuals and though common statements may be made about what is seen, what is seen is seen differently in a geometrical sense. When this observation is extended to a child not only is his external world a much bigger place than an adult's, but it changes from one year to the next as he grows (Figure 1). In addition the adult has a fund of experience to draw on for comparisons, but this is based ultimately on stable relative dimensions.

Therefore, it is very easy for the adult in his fixed situation to make wrong interpretations of what problems a child may face and not to make enough allowances for the adaptability during growth without which a child would be gravely handicapped. This adaptability, though physiologically an essential quality, leads to strange secondary effects that are mostly beneficial but sometimes troublesome in the presence of abnormality, as we shall see. The period of rapid changes in the individual's physique relative to the world around slows down more or less progressively as growth ceases. Therefore, what might be called the need to adapt diminishes and the acquisition and control of essential physical skills has mostly been achieved by late adolescence. In so far as sensation and perception serve these processes, they are dealing with a changing problem and must somehow be included with similar adjustments to the body they inhabit and with the need to contribute eventually to a fully organized, skilled organism.

The demands on the system differ with the needs of the more

or less immobile infant, the tentative gropings and the early slow-motion movements going on to full rapid movement – with visuomotor activity becoming increasingly intricate and controlled. In addition to these developments in what is a flexible situation decided by nature are the demands of the civilized activities of education, sport and speech. The challenge the infant faces, therefore, is to develop – from what is probably a blank sheet of potential vision at birth – a fully functioning system so accurate in input that it can control both motor and perceptive response. These responses have to be made in a changing physical intrinsic environment and have to answer continuously changing needs to understand visually the external world. Whatever he may be born with it is inconceivable that his final performance is ready made.

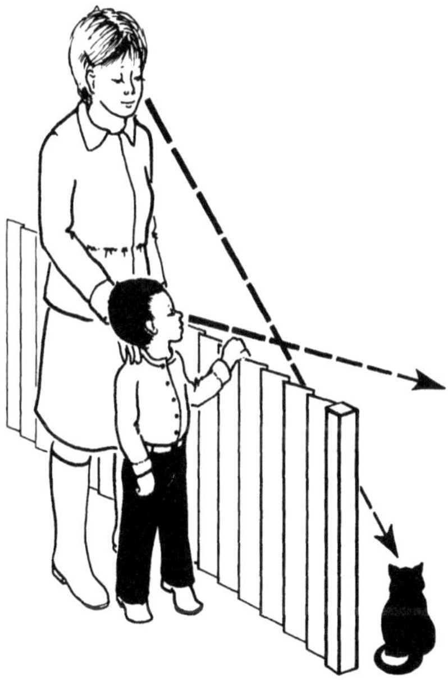

Figure 1 Changing visual opportunity during growth

The study of an infant's visual development must therefore start with a description of what he is born with, the use he appears to make of his equipment and the way in which future demands may be provided for. It must also include a description of the hazards which will interrupt progress towards a perfect visual performance.

A finer discrimination must also be thought of. This is the difference between looking and seeing. Seeing implies some sort of recognition of the meaning of a visual stimulus analogous to the point in an argument reached when it is possible to say 'I see your point'. Our bureaucrats often try to impress by stating they are taking a 'long, hard look at a problem', which indicates no understanding whatever at that stage. Most of us have experienced not seeing an object we are looking at. So although it is difficult to see without looking, it is comparatively easy to look without seeing. This is particularly evident in pictures that are intentionally confusing (Figure 2(a)). These difficulties can be three-dimensional, as in the childrens' game of 'hunt the thimble', which has made many a child wonder why he couldn't see what he was looking at.

Another aspect of visual development is its timing. Other developmental stages are customarily and correctly thought of as being reached over a span of time. Thus many infants walk by the age of one, but many wait twice as long. The same applies to the acquisition of speech and in later years there are big discrepancies in the ages at which reading and writing are achieved. No precise date applies to all children; this should be regarded as normal. It is difficult to be precise about the special senses, and though it is conceivable that even at birth the eye can record the impression of a pinhead accurately, the translation of this into useful vision is altogether different and it takes some years before a child realizes that the moon is not just outside the window (Figure 2(b)). An adult knows the answer, but in a young child anything is possible. Acuity is one thing, useful vision another.

There is considerable controversy over acuity itself in the

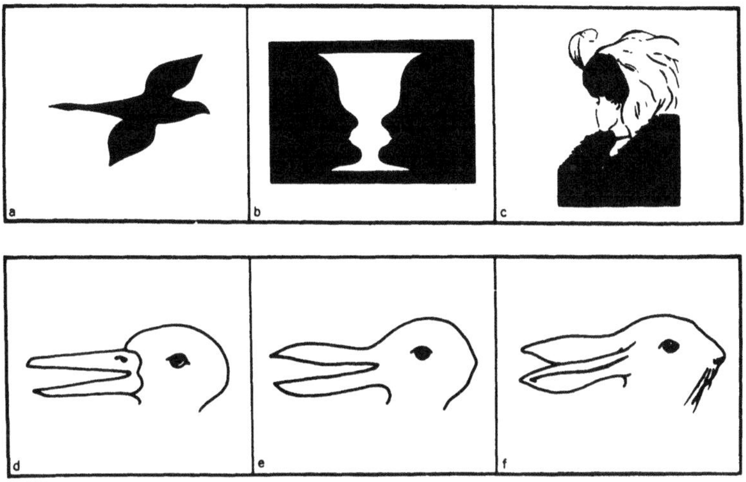

Figure 2(a) Perceptual dilemmas: (a) hawk/goose; (b) vase/faces; (c) girl/crone; (d)–(f) duck/rabbit series [from Frisby, J.P. (1979), *Seeing*. (Oxford University Press) by kind permission]

infant and probably the total visual process must be learnt. If so, the exact timing of each stage will vary. One important characteristic of a learning process is that it is more easily achieved at certain ages than others. For example, the basic skill of speech and language is learnt by children 'naturally' in infancy, even to the extent of their becoming bilingual in some households. Language learning in older children is no longer as natural and easy and it becomes progressively harder to learn a language without study, if not impossible, the later in life the attempt is made. On the other hand, some skills cannot be acquired without preliminary learning of the framework. For most people, all but the simplest mathematics depend on learning the meaning of symbols first, i.e. the ability to read formulae and numbers. Progress towards the higher skill is based on a lower one, which must take time that will vary from person to person. For some the time needed is so long that, as with learning a foreign language, the most favourable time or perhaps the only possible time passes irrevocably. There is evidence that visual development also has its natural stages and that if a natural stage is not achieved during various periods of childhood it never will be[1-4]. This is better expressed by Wordsworth (see page 15). This includes the important ability

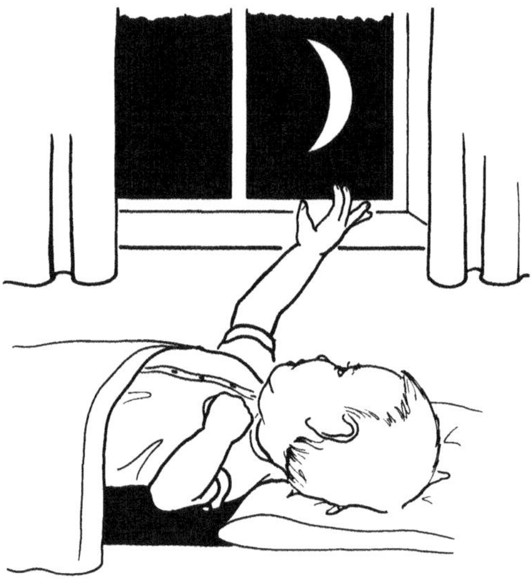

Figure 2(b) How far away is the moon? Within reach? Just out of reach?

to suppress confusing stimuli. We shall see when discussing squints how useful this ability is to the infant and how handicapping its loss becomes in middle childhood – a loss which is afterwards lifelong. This knowledge of the critical stages of natural development colours in a special way the treatment of children for visual defects and necessitates an approach quite different from one suitable for adults.

References

1. Van Hof-Van Duin, J. (1979). Development of visuomotor behaviour in normal and light-deprived cats. In Smith, V. and Keen, J. (eds.) *Visual Handicap in Children.* (*Clinics in Developmental Medicine* No. 73) (London: S.I.M.P. with Heinemann Medical)

2. Blackemore, C. (1974). Development of functional connexions in the mammalian visual system. *B. Med. Bull.*, **30**, 152–157

3. Van Sluyters, R.C. (1974). Reversal of the physiological effects of monocular deprivation in kittens. Further evidence for a sensitive period. *J. Physiol.*, **237**, 195–216

4. Ingram, R.M. (1979). A critical period in the development of squint and amblyopia. In Smith, V. and Keen, J. (eds.) *Visual Handicap in Children.* (*Clinics in Developmental Medicine* No. 73) (London: S.I.M.P. with Heinemann Medical)

Chapter 2

STRUCTURE AND FUNCTION OF THE VISUAL SYSTEM

Detailed knowledge of the structures and linkages of vision is unnecessary, but it is helpful to know the important elements making up the framework.

The fully developed, normally functioning eye is an optical system in principle similar to a camera. Light rays from exterior objects are focused on to a light-sensitive tissue. As in a camera, the light-sensitive structure, in this case the retina, is approached through entirely transparent media with measurable optical quantities. Figure 3 illustrates quite a degree of similarity between the optical arrangements of the eye and the camera. The retinal image is transmitted to the brain as electrical impulses for development. The eye is therefore an organ which assists sight but cannot complete the process. Any defect in transparency will affect transmission and the optical system must be geometrically precise in terms of curvature, intervening distances, thickness, and refractive index.

The light-sensitive cells of the retina consist of rods and cones. The rods in the main are congregated round the periphery of the retina and sensitive to low levels of illumination. The cones are largely assembled in the central area of the retina at the posterior pole, covering some 5–6 mm in diameter. The central portion of this area becomes sharply thinner than its surrounds and is known as the fovea. Here there is an entirely rod-free area with a diameter of about 0.5 mm. Estimates indicate that there are about 2500 cones in this area and some 25 000 over the whole fovea. These cells are those giving a response in good light and to colour. The areas are so small that in clinical medicine the terms fovea, macula and posterior pole are often used loosely and interchangeably to indicate where a lesion is placed. By implication even small lesions affect a large number of cones, leading to a corresponding impairment of detailed vision.

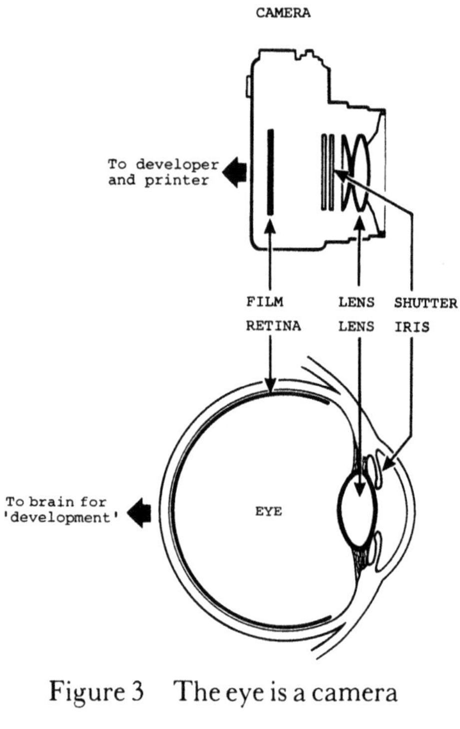

Figure 3 The eye is a camera

The macular area also differs from the rest of the retina in that the retinal vessels do not traverse it, its nutrition being derived from the choroid. This is a mainly vascular covering outside the retina and is covered in its turn by the protective fibrous coat of the sclera.

The nutrition of the avascular cornea is maintained by the

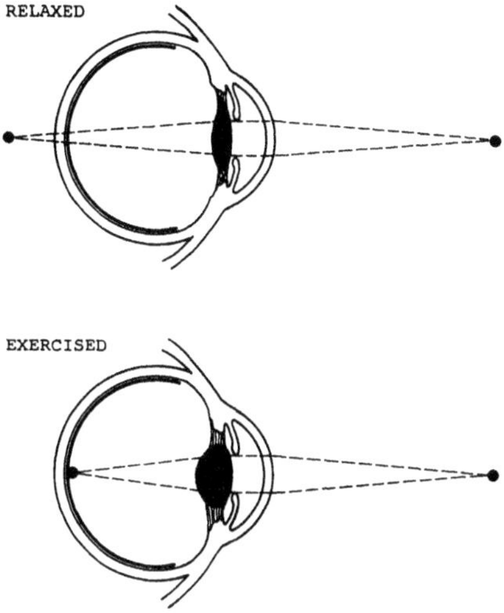

Figure 4 Accommodation: the action of the ciliary muscle on the lens. The increase of the anteroposterior dimension of the lens brings forward the focused image which would otherwise be behind the retina

highly specialized anterior extension of the choroid, the secretory part of the ciliary body. This is responsible for secretion of the aqueous fluid which fills the globe anterior to the lens and maintains a relatively constant intraocular pressure. The ciliary body also has a muscular component which modifies the anteroposterior diameter of the lens and provides a focusing mechanism which enables images of objects at varying distances to be accurately imprinted on the retina (Figure 4).

The iris, in the centre of which is the pupil, is the choroidal layer's most anterior structure. The three elements – choroid, ciliary body and iris – constitute what is called the uvea.

This visual system is mobile. The extraocular muscles which perform the movements are attached to various points in the orbit and are inserted into the sclera. They have unique features because though they are striated like voluntary skeletal muscle, they are more profusely innervated, the muscle fibres are finer than elsewhere and their reactions to choline, acetyl choline and nicotine are anomalous. The significance of these differences is obscure but it is reasonable to suppose that it must be related to the need for precision, rapidity and fine co-ordination in their action.

The control of these muscles by the 3rd, 4th and 6th nerves is ultimately linked intracranially with the corresponding innervation of the synergist muscle of the fellow eye which co-ordinates the movements for binocularity.

The 3rd nerve also carries fibres responsible both for constricting the pupil and for activating the ciliary muscle in accommodation and the convergence element essential if both eyes are to fix on near objects. It is governed, as is the whole near response, by supranuclear connections.

The visual pathway posterior to the retina is via the optic nerve to the optic chiasma, where decussation takes place which ensures that corresponding areas of each retina are represented together on the appropriate side of the brain (the occipital cortex). Relays take place in the retina itself and in the external geniculate bodies. There is ample opportunity in this long traverse for communications with vestibular mechanisms and for all forms of visuomotor responses not only to the eyes, but for head and neck control and co-ordination of physical and somatic responses to visual stimuli whether reflex or voluntary.

The cortex itself can be identified by the naked eye by the arrangement of the white line in the grey matter, which does not occur elsewhere. There is much contemporary controversy concerning the precise function of the cortex. It must be concerned with light sense, colour sense, binocular fusion of the individual images from each eye, perception of form and localization in space.

The eye develops in a complicated way from the primitive differentiation of ectoderm and mesoderm. The forerunner in the embryo is the primary optic vesicle, in which an outgrowth of the forebrain neural ectoderm in contact with surface ectoderm invaginates. The tissue uniting these two layers eventually forms the lens. The lens is therefore derived from surface ectoderm but the retina and optic nerve lying posteriorly from neural ectoderm. The vitreous also has its primitive origin in surface ectoderm. Mesoderm penetrates into this complex as the forerunner of the sclera, the cornea (except for its epithelium), the ciliary muscle, the extrinsic eye muscles and the iris stroma, but not, as one would expect, the iris musculature. Both the sphincter and the dilator of the pupil are unlike any other muscle structure in the body, except the arrectores pilorum, in being derived from ectoderm. This association may seem strange, but it may explain why a frightening sight is commonly said to make hair stand on end. It is also an illustration of how primitive is the reaction to light in the human, compared embryologically and developmentally to that of an organism like hydra.

There are some points in intrauterine growth which may have relevance to postnatal visual development. The retina is in an active stage of development between 28 and 36 weeks but the macular area has lagged behind by 32 weeks and is not fully developed until at least 4 months after birth. This is conceivably a variable delay and in an unknown proportion may be delayed even further. In particular, the cones at birth are short and ill developed, increasing both in length and numbers subsequently. This fact could present an organic structural limit on the visual performance at birth and possibly accounts for the wandering eyes of the infant as well as for the periods of contemplative staring which many normal children exhibit. These considerations may apply even more forcefully to the premature child.

Another feature of retinal development which is completed only at birth is the myelination of the nerve fibres from the ganglion cells which have penetrated the brain. Myelination begins posteriorly and reaches the nerve head only at birth, probably not being complete even then.

Myelination of the higher visual pathways is also incomplete and is only beginning in the association tracts. Again 4 months is stated to be the period before the process is completed. Whether this delay interferes with full function and in what way is debatable, but must be taken into account in theorizing about early visual capacity. Postnatal development is not confined to these neural elements and in fact the lens, though fully functional as an optical mechanism at birth, continues to grow throughout life, mainly anteroposteriorly, its transparent fibres being laid on top of one another as in an onion.

Amongst other anomalies which may be present at birth and which may have an intrauterine cause is a persistent pupillary membrane. This is a filamentary network of ghost vessels which have not fully atrophied. The fetal eye is a highly vascular tissue and the visual pathway has to be clear of vessels before the eye can achieve full transparency. It is thought that the break-up of the vasculature of the vitreous may be responsible for the specks which most people see looking at a bright surface, known to the ophthalmologist as muscae volitantes.

The sclera develops from aggregations of tissue near the insertion of the recti muscles and the posterior part is the last to form. In high myopia the posterior sclera in particular is thinner and expanded out of proportion to the rest of the globe. One of the many hypotheses put forward to explain congenital myopia rests on this developmental fact.

Accommodation will be discussed later, but developmentally the ciliary muscle responsible for its operation continues to change after birth and is said by one authority[1] not to reach adult dimensions until the age of 18. Because hypermetropic eyes require an over-exertion of accommodation for all accurate vision and normal eyes cannot see near objects without accommodating, these changes may be very important.

Another prolonged postnatal process is the elaboration of the iris stroma. Its complete architecture takes several years to develop and is said by some to be as individual in pattern eventually as fingerprints. There is no known scientific foundation for the cult of 'augendiagnose' of systemic disease by the study of iris patterns, and this prolonged process of change in the pattern from its comparatively simple appearance at birth must make paediatric medicine difficult for practitioners of the art.

Aristotle noted that all white-skinned babies have blue eyes at birth. Pigmentation appears in many in the first few days of life. The complex process of pigmentation throughout the body is only partially understood and apart from albinism in its various forms, the colour of the eyes has little relevance to visual performance. For the paediatrician the condition known as anisochromia (different-coloured eyes) may be important in an individual. In the adult depigmentation of the iris may occur in Horner's syndrome leading to different coloured eyes. In the infant the same disorder may lead to failure of one eye to pigment. Horner's syndrome (ptosis, miosis and enophthalmos) is caused by disturbance of the cervical sympathetic system, sometimes associated with a disparity of accommodation between the two eyes. Rarely it can arise from congenital deformities at the lung apex. Difference in iris pigmentation is not caused by genetic mixture and other causes should be looked for.

The position at birth can be summarized as incomplete in the following respects:

(1) Lack of retinal pigment.
(2) Macula undifferentiated.
(3) Incomplete myelination of higher centres.
(4) The ciliary muscle is relatively undeveloped.
(5) The dilator pupillae is weak.
(6) The iris pigment is underdeveloped.

Most of these are thought to complete their development in the first few months, though development of the ciliary muscle, the iris pigment and its dilator muscle are further delayed. The dilator pupillae in particular is said to take several years.

These facts imply that the functions performed in the fully developed eye are not likely to be available to the infant. The immature macula and the lack of myelination would almost certainly be a barrier to precise vision, including perhaps colour vision.

The lack of retinal pigment and the poor density of iris pigment could presumably influence the appreciation of changes in illumination, which could also be affected by the weakness of the dilator muscle of the pupil. The small pupil which is the rule in infancy could be a protective mechanism. In addition, were it not for the small pupil in early infancy the developing retina might be injured by high intensities of illumination. One of the major changes presented to the infant on emergence from the darkness of the womb must be exposure to light. This appears to be a striking example of the adaptability of infants; as far as is known no intraocular damage occurs from this cause.

The immaturity of important elements and the theoretical difficulty of assuming that there can be any ordered cognitive ability at birth leads to the conclusion that at this stage only the ground plan of future visual competence is present. This conclusion receives support from studying visual behaviour in the cradle.

Reference

1. Stieve, R. (1963). Quoted by Weale, R.A., *The Ageing Eye*. (H.K. Lewis)

Chapter 3

VISION IN EARLY CHILDHOOD

The interpretation of the visual performance of infants and even of older children by outsiders is difficult and many mistakes are made, either by over- or underestimation. Odd head postures, squints and retardation are often assumed to mean a poor or substandard visual performance, though when measured the acuity is normal. On the other hand, formal testing of an overall normality of visual behaviour may, for instance, unmask one blind eye. Though this situation from birth is not as serious as might be thought, ignorance of the fact that only one eye is useful is professional failure on the part of doctors.

Although there is great variability in visual behaviour and performance throughout childhood, there are important stages of development which must be recognized and recorded by paediatricians whatever their timing.

The following description of the stages of the development of visual behaviour is only a guide, but marked divergences from the normal pattern are sufficient danger signals to merit ophthalmological advice. In those families with known serious visual defects of early onset advice is desirable if only to reassure the parents that all is well. These children need careful and more frequent observation than those with a normal visual heredity as there is a higher prevalence of defect amongst them.

In all observations and testing procedures which guide judgements the presence of a response properly comprehended is a much more valuable sign than its absence. Throughout childhood there is the difficulty of distinguishing between what a child cannot do and what he appears not to be interested in doing or won't do. One positive achievement indicates what can be done; one failure to achieve may well be due to any number of extraneous factors which may have no relevance to the faculty being examined.

STAGES IN NORMAL CHILDREN[1]

Up to 4 weeks

Response to light sources are present. The pupils must respond to light shone from a torch in twilight or darkness. Failure to do this requires immediate attention. Eyes and head turn towards a window, for example, and linger if the child's body is slowly turned away from such a stimulus. Similarly, an attempt to follow near and large objects can be seen, notably the mother's face. This type of response can be obtained by simulation with pendulum-type testing with bright balls swung slowly up to 45 cm (18 in) distance from the child's face[2]. There are other possible responses which indicate visual interest, notably blinking when a sudden bright light is shone on the eyes whether or not attempts are made to fix the eyes upon it.

Lid closure rather than fixation may be the response to torchlight stimulus. This is normal and not a pathological photophobia, though if it is persistent and carried over into dislike of normal ambient lighting it may sometimes indicate abnormalities such as aniridia or buphthalmos.

The test should be performed on each eye separately with scrupulous care that the stimulus is strictly confined to the eye being examined. One normal eye is enough for excellent vision so that whatever may be the cause of a failure to respond in one eye and important as it is to find it, talk of blindness is a mistake at this stage.

Difficulties occasionally arise because of the small size of the infant pupil. This can be overcome by using a magnifier. The failure to respond is of less importance visually if other positive visual responses are present, but ophthalmological interpretation is still desirable.

These anomalies are much more likely to occur in infants with other abnormalities than in otherwise completely healthy and normal children.

It is stated by many observers that eye-to-eye gaze is the predominant visual activity of the infant, which may possibly be broadened to interest in the face. This idea is pursued by some to the length of stating that a two-dimensional caricature of a face is always a good and interesting substitute for a three-dimensional reality (Figure 5). The sophistication required to see the representational similarity, on a commonsense view,

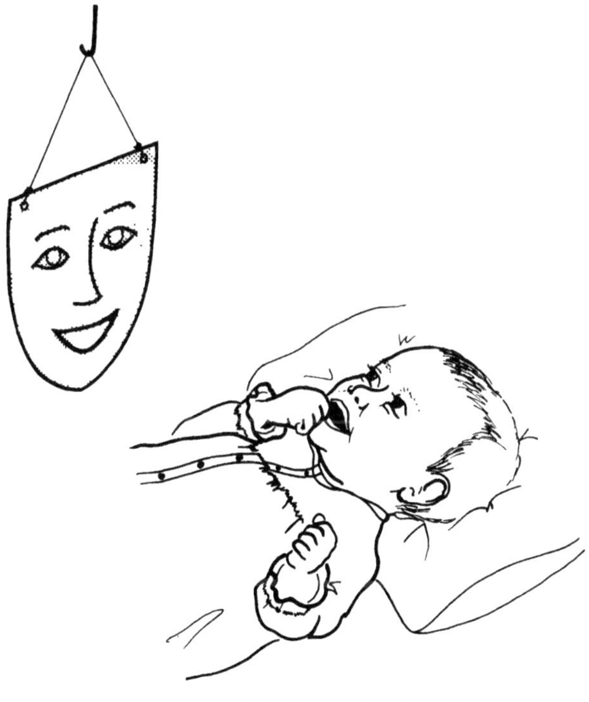

Figure 5 Mother substitute?

seems too extreme to be reliable. On the other hand, the mother's face and also intermittent interference by anyone in the general field of vision of the infant should stimulate some sort of response. The additional stimulus provided by sounds emerging from the visual stimulus will give an extra lead to initial interest, but may be misleading without careful interpretation. The definitive stimulus must be silent. Handheld mirrors often provide the infant with a visual impression interesting enough to fix on if only momentarily. Toys incorporating a mirror can be found but are not easily obtained from medical and optical sources.

Such eye movements as occur are disjointed and erratic, though by the age of a month when the child is held upright and when nothing near to the face is available, rudimentary searching and scanning further afield begins to be noticeable.

1–3 Months

At this age a baby starts to be extremely interested in his own finger play and spends time with the eyes converging on to them in front of his face. He will also become more consistent and persistent in attempts to follow a ball dangled at a distance of, say, 15–25 cm (6–10 in). These visual activities are directed mostly at near objects. The lids close protectively if a hand is rapidly moved across the field of vision at about 5 cm (2 in) distance. This is not necessarily a visual response, because babies can be sensitive to the draught which may be produced or to a light touch which can occur in this exercise.

3–6 Months

The infant's visual interest is still mainly restricted to objects which might be within his reach, though if these objects are mobile he will extend his observation much further afield for larger ones, such as people or animals.

Elementary visuomotor activities, such as foot grasping and

attempts to touch and pick up objects of all sizes within range, begin to be elaborated.

All these activities seem to indicate that visual experience is built up on events close at hand and that distance vision is superimposed on this as the infant progresses toward being mobile and therefore being able to plan a route towards something desirable or to avoid an obstruction which might be harmful.

It is therefore necessary for the paediatrician to forget the ophthalmological custom of quoting distance vision as the primary measure of acuity, whereas it is really the ultimate.

To a certain extent the environment of a child in the cradle is self-sufficient visually; but those who hope for a child of versatility should not be reluctant to give him varied opportunities with 'mobiles' from time to time and new toys to study and handle.

The evaluation of an infant's vision as opposed to its apparatus is therefore largely based on informally noting that the activities described are present and roughly on time. Delay or anomalous behaviour, particularly in children who are delayed in other respects, indicates a need for a formal ophthalmic opinion and continued watchfulness even where no organic abnormality is detected.

SIMPLE TESTS IN INFANCY AND EARLY CHILDHOOD

Orthoptists were trained to deal with squints by methods that encouraged co-ordinated eye movements and the use of binocular mechanisms. This led to extensive exploration of the meaning of children's visual responses, so the orthoptist's activities expanded to include more detailed investigation. For this reason they constitute, largely untapped, a body of high expertise in testing visual function in young children in the UK. It is only recently that this has been recognized and though projects have been successfully mounted which demonstrate their ability to detect visual defects in child population screening programmes, these are isolated and have yet to be given their full value and to be organized by the National Health Service as part of the preventive services. The following is a modification of a battery of tests quoted by Mclellan[3].

(1) Pen torch – fixation and movements. Pupil reaction, symmetry and clarity, corneal reflections.
(2) Cover test for near and distance vision.
(3) Ocular movements.
(4) Prism bar.
(5) Catford drum (opticokinetic nystagmus).
(6) Rolling balls (Stycar) and Hundreds and Thousands.
(7) Sheridan Gardiner, Beale Collins.
(8) Stycar toys.
(9) Money.
(10) Keys.
(11) Sweets.
(12) Titmus Stereo test.

These tests are an attempt to systematize and supplement the impressions obtained by casual observation of visual behaviour and the younger the child the more they can be open to misinterpretation. This is particularly likely when failure to perform a test is noticed. Success has greater significance than failure. The reasons for failure may be lack of attention, lack of rapport, unsuitable environment, fright, fatigue, hunger, thirst, indigestion, and in older children a full bladder from organic or psychological sources.

The environment

This plays a large part in a successful examination. The best arrangement is a totally simple one in the examination room. There should be a minimum of diversions such as pictures, toys and gadgets. All of the child's attention is needed by the examiner. For this reason any assistant needs to be well trained and unobtrusive, to avoid being not only a diversionary visual attraction but also a noisy one. Unplanned movements about the room are sure to catch the child's eye at times and sounds such as taps running, the telephone or knocks on the door are often the end of a promising manoeuvre.

The ideal team for most testing consists of the examiner, the parent and the child. The presence of siblings will nearly always sabotage testing. Intermittent noises, such as a busy road near by or the sudden wailing of an ambulance siren, will overwhelm carefully constructed schemes of testing. The room can be large or small, but should not lose a homely atmosphere. The examiner should be the only interesting or the dominating figure of interest in the room. It helps rapport if the examiner wears conventional clothing, particularly avoiding a white coat which quite young children associate with real or imaginary unpleasantness.

All these tests require co-operation in varying degrees and great difficulties arise in children who are frightened or resentful. Clinical inspection of the eyes, though not acuity testing, can be greatly helped in infants by quietening with a sugared teat or finger or bottle, and some young children feel more secure and will give more attention if they are supported on the mother's shoulder with the examiner behind rather than in front of her.

The interpretation of the visual response in infants is differently based from that in older children who can express what they see in words. Interpretation depends largely on observing fixation, following movements by the eyes and responses to stimuli by the child reaching or pointing. Fixation may or may not be real and its value depends on the stimulus. Fixation on to a light and following it is of positive value, but if there is failure to follow it becomes difficult to be certain whether the initial fixation was coincidental.

Among significant responses in quite young infants are smiling, frowning, jumping, eye closure, head turning on stimulation, and any gesture; but again the absence of these is not definite evidence that the visual response is defective. However, if no positive responses are elicited or if the visual behaviour of a child indicates the possibility of an abnormality the situation becomes an ophthalmological one, particularly if there is any family history of infantile visual disorders.

Since a child's visual behaviour and general development will be quite normal with one blind or severely defective eye, testing should, ideally, be performed on each eye separately. Infants and young children, however, seldom tolerate covering of one eye more than momentarily and the irritation or resentment caused by the cover usually spoils general rapport for a time as well as preventing successful monocular testing. If their resentment of covering is more marked in one eye than the other then this is a strong indication that only one eye has defective vision.

Hence all tests of acuity or response in young children need to be repeated at intervals if they have been equivocal or inexplicably negative. Any findings must be related to the child's visual behaviour both in general and in the examination room. Visual behaviour and general activity may often be normal, whereas the performance of tests to demand would indicate quite poor visual ability. This is particularly the case in children suffering from brain damage.

Notes on tests

Torch. Inspecting the reaction of the pupil to light gives valuable information. Constriction indicates intact light-sensitive pathways. Failure to constrict may indicate defective light sense or have a neurological cause, but beware of it being the result of recent dilatation for the purposes of examining the media and fundi. In all cases of an absent or sluggish pupillary response the cause must be searched for. Secondly, a torch is a mobile source of light and the eye movements can be studied as the child follows it. Thirdly, the light is reflected off each cornea symmetrically. This reflection is central when the eyes are being used for distant objects and off centre by an equal amount in a temporal direction in each eye when they are convergent for near vision. This observation in very young children or uncooperative children is extremely difficult to make except at close range. Asymmetry of this reflex indicates a squint, but care must be taken that the torch is midline. When using a torch for light response it is important to avoid clicking the switch as the infant may respond to the sound rather than to the light. This test for a squint, like the cover test which follows, is not always easy to interpret, because of the reasons described below.

The cover test. The normal position of each eye when fixing an object is symmetrical against a vertical or horizontal plane. This can be expressed as stating that unless a squint is present both eyes are looking at the same object. Therefore, covering first one eye and then the other while the child fixes an object should produce no movement at the moment of fixation. This is not an easy test to interpret in an infant, especially for distance. The difficulty is to be sure that the child is fixing the object in the first place and then does not lose it by inattention or confusion when the second eye is uncovered or occluded in its turn. The child's natural interest is in the object nearest his eye, i.e. the occluder and not in the object the examiner holds. Therefore, when the occluder is moved he will often either attempt to see where it has gone or lose interest. In either case haphazard movements of the eyes may occur which defeat the purpose of the test. In the case of loss of interest no movement may occur, even though the eye is squinting. A 10° squint or even smaller is pathological, so the movement being watched for is also small. None the less this is an excellent test if its difficulties are overcome and consistent results obtained.

Ocular movements. A possible false finding, apart from those caused by inattention, is the production of pseudonystagmus by forcing lateral movements beyond normal acceptance.

The prism bar depends on its production of diplopia, either horizontal or vertical. The eyes should make the appropriate movement to overcome the diplopia produced by the prism. This is difficult to interpret under the age of 6 months (before binocular reflexes are expected to be reliable) but consistent results indicate an abnormality requiring further investigation.

Opticokinetic nystagmus is produced by moving alternate black-and-white strips across the field of vision and can be elicited in the infant. Failure, as usual, may not indicate more than visual disinterest.

The Catford drum uses a system of grading these stimuli so that a rough measure of the acuity is possible. A possible criticism is that acuity as measured by a moving object is not strictly comparable with stationary objects; but the measurements are intrinsically comparable and this is therefore a useful tool in very young children.

Rolling balls. The same criticism applies in older children to the use of graded balls rolled at a fixed distance, and once more the element of visual attention plays a great part so that positive results are more significant than negative ones[2].

The Stycar and Sheridan/Gardiner material[1,2,5]. From quite an early age children can match objects if their interest can be aroused and the Stycar material consists of toys and models which provide useful information to the examiner. Although the ability to fix and follow a small rolling ball obviously indicates good acuity, the inability to do so does not mean poor acuity because of the attention factor, but it should herald further ophthalmic investigation. The ability to see moving objects is not as difficult as seeing stationary ones, so although this test is useful normality cannot be claimed until a line of letters (6/6 size) can be read or matched. The same limitation, though to a rather lesser degree, can be put on the interpretation of fixed balls. (Both these tests are part of the Stycar testing material.)

In the third and fourth year of life this ability to match develops so that standard Snellen letters can be used and matched both for near and distance. In addition it becomes progressively easier to test each eye separately. This requires effective occlusion. Possibly the most acceptable occluder in older children is the spring type which fits lightly but completely over the eye, thus eliminating the most common source of error in testing the vision of children, namely peeping through a chink in the occluder. The printed testing material consists in its simplest form of single letters rather than a line. Acuity obtained in this way is usually better, especially when defects are present, than when the letter to be matched is on a line. For comparability and measurement of strict normality the line method gives a more accurate result. In practice the somewhat detailed instructions given for the letter matching, i.e. five- or seven-letter cards, can be ignored. Most children who can match consistently will do so on the seven-letter card and it is quite easy to cover some of these with a sheet of paper if it is suspected that there is some bewilderment of choice.

Every practitioner devises methods which seem helpful to him for vision testing. Amongst these may be the use of coins or a bunch of keys for following movements at various distances. These are useful because most people carry them habitually, so the equipment is always available. Both can attract the child's attention by the noise they make but can be used silently for the operative part of the test once interest has been aroused. Distance vision is much more difficult to grade than near vision in infancy because the immobile infant has no great incentive for interest in something beyond his reach.

Hundreds and Thousands. This is an excellent test of near vision. The brand consisting of the smallest particles is the best to use and fixation on one of these or better still attempts to retrieve indicate normal near vision. Failing Hundreds and Thousands (Figure 6: facing p. 64) any small sweet provides a test of useful near vision.

The above collection of tests is by its nature objective and ignores the subjective element in visual activity except by presumption. However, matching tests have as one of their advantages over naming tests the avoidance of mistakes in naming *per se*.

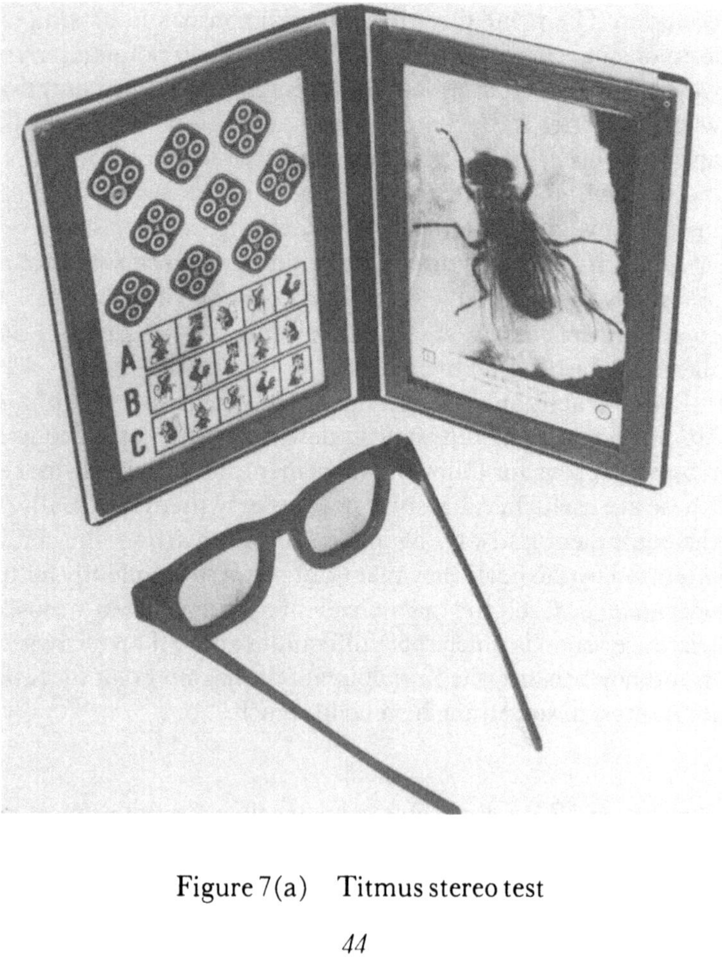

Figure 7(a) Titmus stereo test

Picture tests. Many attempts have been made to construct picture tests to conform with the optical requirements underlying the familiar and universal test type for adults and older children. One in common use is the Beale Collins picture test. This type always fails on two counts. Firstly, there has to be an element of stylization because of the optical requirements and of portraying three-dimensional objects in two dimensions. Secondly, the examiner himself is faced with difficulties if a child calls a chicken a bird or a duck. Similarly, an elephant may be distinguished in this type of test from a cow by the absence of an udder or horns and the presence of a trunk and big ears. However, many children who know about cows may not be so familiar with elephants and may call all four-footed creatures dogs or cows, or even more simply an animal. The result is always difficulty for the examiner.

Titmus Stereo test (Figure 7). This is a time-saving test of binocular vision. Using polarized glasses the flat picture is thrown into relief when binocular vision is present. Though not

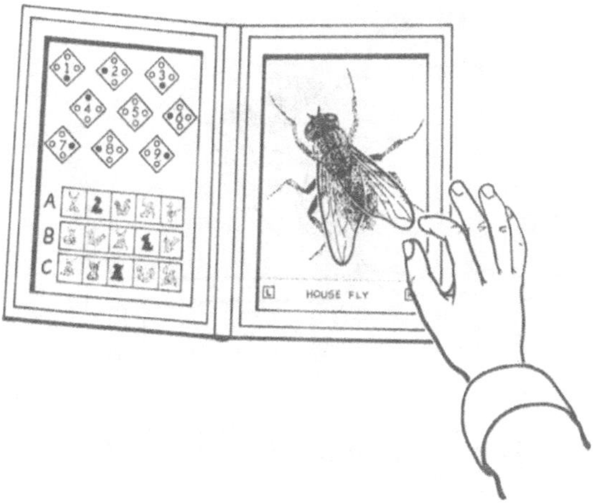

Figure 7(b) When the fly is seen binocularly the wings stand out of the picture and the child will indicate this when he is asked to feel them

fully reliable in children under 5 years a positive result does indicate the presence of binocular depth perception. Negative or equivocal tests are relatively common and should not, in very young children, be the sole indicator for referral.

Other widely used tests now dropping out of universal favour (E test, hand test, Landolt rings) depended on orientating an object to match the position of its copy at 6 m (20 ft). These tests fail not only because a child is not accurate in placing an E in, say, a north or south position so that one may be put NE and the other SE, but he often places it in a different plane altogether so that the E in the vertical plane is, for example, converted into an E in the horizontal plane. Nobody would claim that this is how the child sees vertical objects. Whether he does or not the interpretation is a spatial one rather than a guide to acuity (Figure 8).

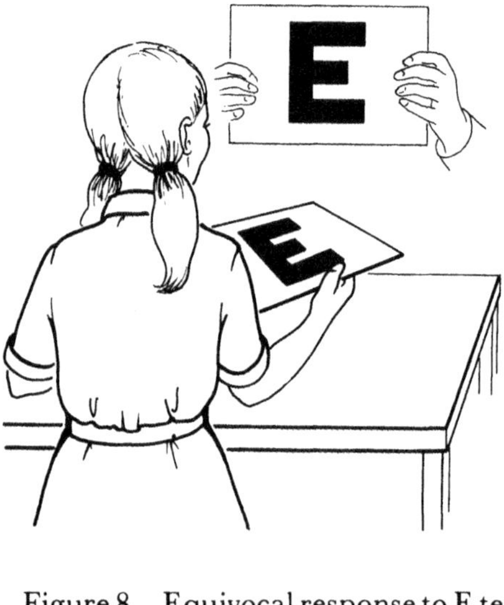

Figure 8 Equivocal response to E test

Dr Mary Sheridan was the pioneer in exposing the faults in these tests which held the field when, as a paediatrician, she tried to relate ophthalmic practice to the realities of clinical testing of young children in paediatric clinics. It is to her that we owe the revolution in the methods of testing infants and young children now accepted by ophthalmologists themselves in daily practice.

Until children are fully and reliably literate matching tests have a reasonably accurate role, provided they are ultimately done on a linear basis. Their use as single type is less accurate but enables comparison between eyes and at intervals of time in co-operative children.

Near vision can also be tested by matching methods. Changes in near vision can indicate increasing retinal discrimination in the treatment of squints, often antedating improvement in distance vision so that its measurement is a help to orthoptists as well as to those responsible for relating school performance to visual ability or potential.

Experience shows that children are less inclined to remain interested in tests for detailed distance vision than similar tests for near vision. In both cases the analysis of a line is more difficult for them, possibly for perceptual reasons rather than visual.

It is often wrongly assumed that children need large print for visual reasons when they learn to read, but again the reasons are perceptual. An interesting experiment relating to this was performed at a Borstal Institution for adolescents. Large-print books were mixed with normal-print books with similar titles and contents in the library. The books in large print were used far more often than those with normal print despite being more cumbersome.

It is difficult to standardize the distance of the material when testing near vision and in younger children better not to try. The smallest print read should be recorded and the distance chosen by the child. If a reliable test can be done at about 25 cm (10 in) this should be added to the report (see Table 1, p. 72).

Near vision may be recorded as N*x* in ophthalmological reports. The following show an approximation to print sizes in common use:

N 4.5 – Small advertisements, the *Radio Times*, footnotes.
N 5 – Telephone directory.
N 6 – Small newsprint.
N 8 – Average newspaper.
N 12 – Large typescript.
N 18 – Small headlines, large-print books.
N 36 – Large headlines.

In many of the physiological or more particularly psychological tests of visual function and perception much is made of eye dominance. Ophthalmologists recognize that most people have a preferred eye and that this preference is settled early in life, but in general clinical practice it seems to have no influence on function unless, as is often the case, it is preferred because its acuity is better than its partner's. Anomalies of laterality and their relation to eye dominance have become matters to study in relation to visual perception, but seldom quote the refraction or acuity. This being so it seems better for the average clinician not engaged in research to concentrate on the preferred eye and the ocular reasons for it (which could be a squint as well as a refractive disorder) rather than look for more deep-seated, central and perceptual connotations.

AN EXAMPLE OF TESTING

Every child needs a different approach by the examiner and each child will not necessarily follow his previous pattern. A note such as 'very unco-operative' for a child aged 2 years should not ring alarm signals about his performance at 4 years and there is no need to be apprehensive. Exactly the same can happen in reverse. A docile child of 2 may become a scared, revolutionary 4-year-old.

It is therefore pointless to try to rehearse every possible event. For this reason the testing procedure of an immediate pre-school child has been chosen because it should be possible at this age to get accurate results comparable with adult vision (with reservations). At earlier ages testing has to be modified so much to allow for the child's immaturity that it prevents a full programme, which will contain all the elements for confidence in all the aspects required. Testing at younger ages is aimed at discovering defects rather than recording substantive acuity which will be lasting, though it often does produce a useful basic record, if the principle already laid down that a positive result carries more certainty than a negative one is observed.

The atmosphere

A child of 5 years is very sophisticated and knows the ways of the world. If you are dressed in a certain way you have characteristics which he thinks he can recognize as all sophisticated people do. Many mothers will have briefed the child on what to expect and may have used phrases like 'blacking out one eye', which suggests some form of mutilation.

The atmosphere needs to be as normal and casual as possible so that the child does not sense anything resembling a medical where his clothes come off or injections are a possibility. Therefore, white coats are to be avoided. This build-up is not entirely for the child's benefit but is aimed at achieving a quick and accurate test. A reluctant or distracted child is not likely to provide this. If possible, siblings should be elsewhere. Those that mean to be helpful are sometimes more interfering than those who are uninterested. This also applies to some mothers and if the child can bear to sit on his own with his mother a little way off this is a suitable arrangement. It is good practice for the mother to be able to see what is going on.

While the preliminaries are being attended to it is as well to ask the mother whether the child has ever had an eye test – and if so why, when and where. Further questioning depends a little on whether the examination is for screening or because there is already a possible visual problem. For screening there is mainly the question of family history. Most mothers consider only themselves and their children to be the family; a few include their husbands. It pays to be more specific about any troubles in childhood of both parents' siblings and parents. If two visits are made additional pieces of relevant information are commonly added on the second visit.

When a complaint is thought to be present the mother will usually begin by describing the particular sign that is troubling. This may be, for example, rubbing the eyes. Questions then asked should include how often the sign occurs, whether on any particular occasion, during any particular visual task or time of day, and so on. The most important questions otherwise are about whether the eyes or lids look abnormal, water, discharge and above all about visual behaviour. Mothers always have an opinion about their child's vision – usually optimistic – and it is always worth asking whether the child prefers to sit close to the television set and how strong the preference is. While all this questioning is taking place the child should be watched closely for pointers and also to size up the chances of a successful examination. Sometimes it relaxes the child to see some rapport appearing between you and his mother. With other children it is better to go straight ahead and defer questioning until afterwards. This is particularly so with younger children.

Matching (Figure 10)

The most important result of the examination is the visual acuity and it is always best to attempt this first of all. Using the Sheridan Gardiner matching material the first step is to give the child 'his' card, ask him to look at it and then at yours as close as he likes with both eyes open. Then tell him that the letter you are showing him is on his card, and ask if he can find it and touch it with his finger. If he is brisk and correct then it is worth trying another for consistency. If all goes well the next move has to be explained, which is either to tell him to wait while you go 6 m (20 ft) away or to show him that you can wave your card and that he can see it in the mirror. Many children find the mirror image more easily if the card is waved before they are asked to match it. Working down from 6/60 each correct response must be given full praise. Some children prefer a challenge and the instructions can be: 'Try this one' – 'now another one' – 'Can you find this one?' – 'I wonder if you can do this very small one, which is the last one.' The full sequence does not have to be done, especially the first time over when it is best done binocularly with an alert co-operative child. Usually 6/36 and one smaller type are enough. It then has to be explained that one eye must be covered: 'Can he do the test again with just one eye?' The spring occluder is a good method in older children (Figure 9), but if this is resisted the mother may be called in to

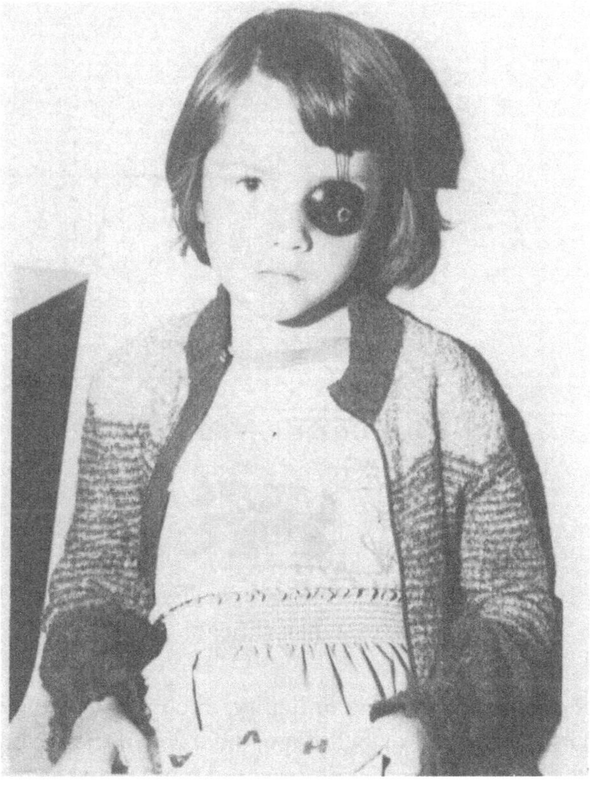

Figure 9 Spring occluder

cover the eye with the palm of her hand making sure there are no chinks. This is often overdone and pressure on the globe is enough to produce a false result when the occluded eye is tested in its turn. It is wise to wait a couple of minutes and to retest the second eye if a defective acuity has been found. There are many

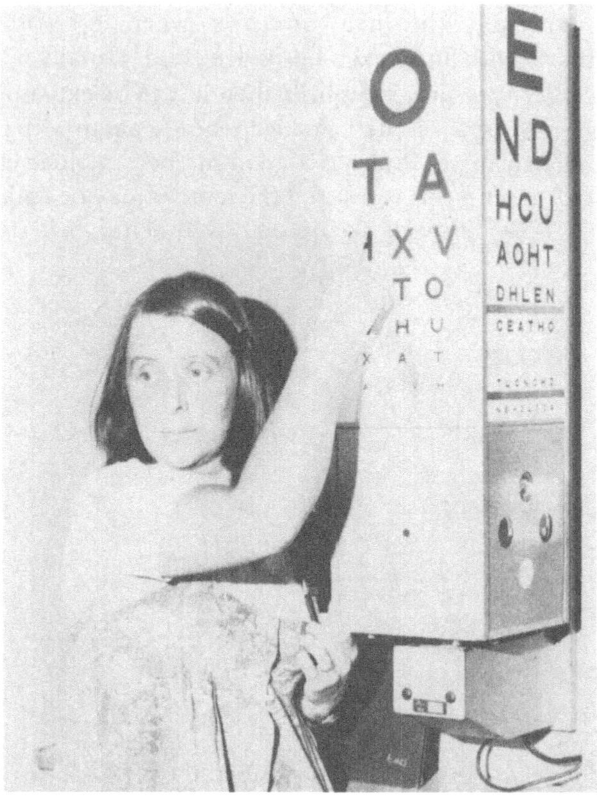

Figure 10 Linear Sheridan–Gardiner Test. (a) The letter to be matched (linear)

ways of getting round this difficulty, such as a piece of gauze fixed with Dermocell or Sellotape, a card or a tissue; but they are time consuming and often resented more than the mother's hand. If the child already wears glasses much the best is a tissue between the eye and the glass on one side and then the other (Figure 10(b) and 11). If the test is being done from 6 m (20 ft) the mother will be needed to verify the match from behind or beside the child.

It often saves time and trouble if the near-vision test is done on each eye immediately after it has been occluded for distance. The child should be allowed to choose his distance for near-vision if he dislikes 25 cm (10 in) and a note made of the distance he demands to identify the smaller letters.

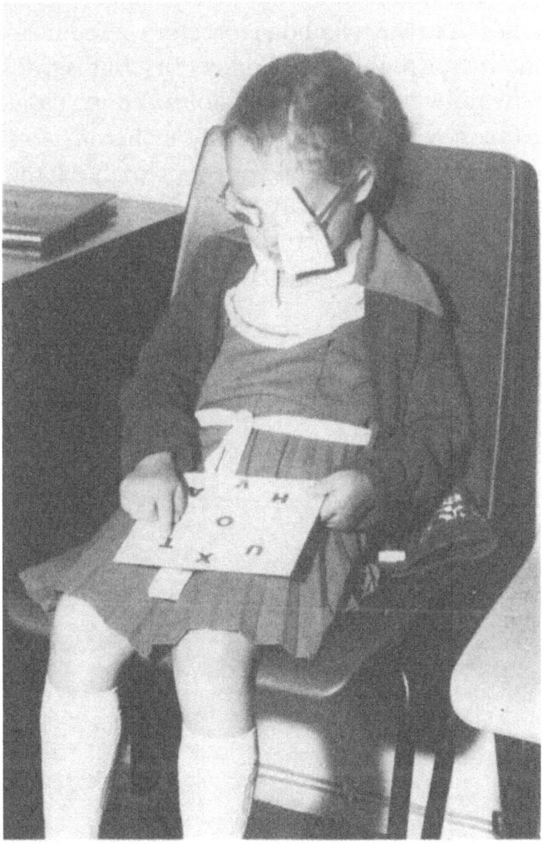

Figure 10(b) The letter to be matched by a child wearing tissue occlusion

Children of school age and before are quite capable of seeing very small print close to and there would be no need for them to start learning with large print were it not for the problem of scanning. The inability to see small print is an indicator of possible visual fatigue occurring in a spell of reading earlier than normal.

The method is for the child to retain his matching card and for the examiner to use a fine pointer (for example a nail file) to indicate the letter to be matched (Figure 11). The best test card to use is the card which gives the 6/6 equivalent, which is type rather smaller than the telephone directory – about N4. This is not a common type found in orthodox tests, but is traditionally used in many railway and bus timetables. Young children who fail to see this type at near, especially if there is a consistent deficiency of one eye only, should be very closely examined for a squint and be reviewed at an interval of not more than 3 months, and then referred for refraction and further advice even if distance acuity is good.

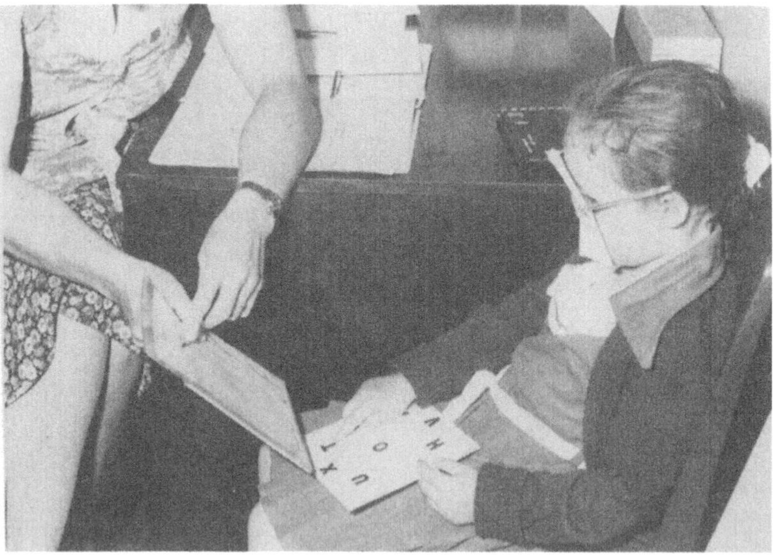

Figure 11 Matching test using a pointer to indicate small print

Near-vision testing by reading words includes disentangling literacy from visual defect (Figure 12). Two popular tests challenge the child with 'lazibones' in the first three words in one instance and with 'camomile' in the other. A good comprehensive test with grading for literacy is the Maclure reading type for children, but this is somewhat elaborate for screening purposes.

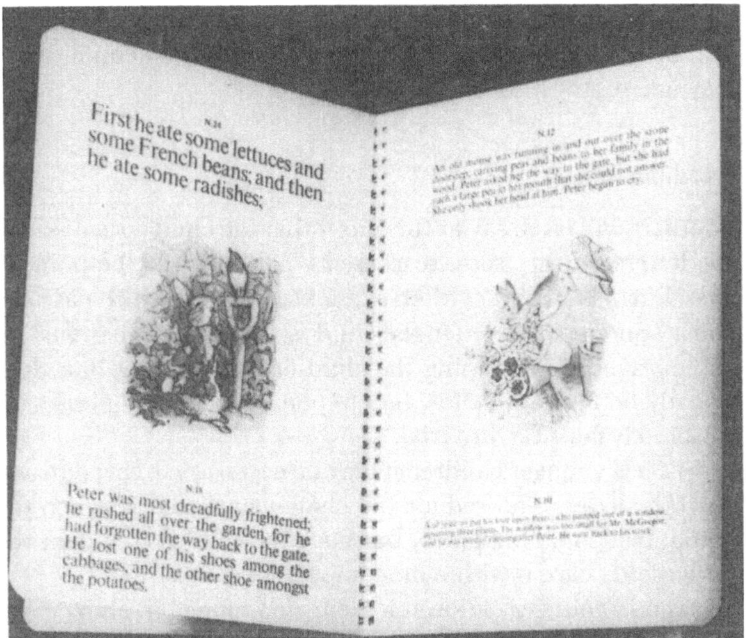

Figure 12 Standard near vision test type [by courtesy of C. Davis Keeler Ltd.]

The partially sighted may be able to read very small print but only at very small distances. This ability may make the critical difference for their place of education. It is a very useful finding, and can be missed if there is an insistence on 25 cm.

A colour-vision test with matching letters follows naturally at this stage, being based on similar principles (Figure 13: facing p. 64). One is 'The Guy's Colour Vision Test for Young or Handicapped Children'[6]. It is better to insist on matching rather than naming the letters, as this avoids an irrelevant source of error. The plates are in no particular order except that the first two are only to establish that the method is understood.

The defective consistently pick out the confusion letter in all the plates. Anything less than this is not likely to have any practical significance and those whose performance is muddled can be left a year or two for confirmation. It is essential to use daylight for the most accurate results.

Modifications

Mothers will often say at the outset that the child doesn't know his letters but are soon reassured when they see the point of matching. The mother often cannot see 6/6, in which case she must announce the letter the child is indicating. She must be discouraged from helping the child or intimidating him. It is usually better not to allow him to name the letters unless he is absolutely faultless on a trial.

In a few younger children it may be necessary to cover up two or three letters and reduce the choice, particularly when the initial trial is taking place; but once the child is confident the seven-letter card is within the competence of most.

Even in younger children it seems too refined in many cases to consider using a smaller number of letters, i.e. five, on the matching card and better to perform the test on an *ad hoc* basis. If a child can match confidently and consistently, which is essential for a sound test, he is usually capable of accurate choice also.

He should not be allowed the occasional mistake once the test proper begins after establishing that he has understood the method. If uncertainty remains and the mistakes are inconsistent with any particular visual level or appear to be due to fatigue a repeat test another day is the next step. At the second examination it is best to go straight for the particular problem which arose the first time.

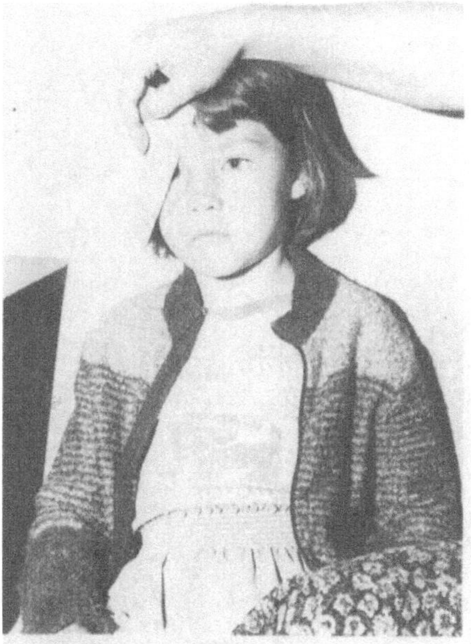

Figure 14(a) Cover test using a card (wrong)

Any child with 6/6 vision in each eye for distance and the equivalent for near will probably not show any serious pathological condition, but eye movements must be tested, i.e. their full excursion right, left, up and down. The cover test should be performed for near and distance vision. Results of the cover test in the distance are often equivocal but if the child is fixing properly on a point of light or a letter at 6 m (20 ft) the covered eye will move when given its turn either inwards or outwards or vertically, depending on the nature of the squint. Beware of covering with the fingers; they are seldom without chinks. A card or envelope tucked into the nose is better (Figure 14(a) and (b)). Arranging the card so that the examiner can see what the covered eye is doing behind it is informative. Gross divergence which straightens so quickly on cover removal that it can easily be missed by a fatigued or inaccurate examiner may thus be detected.

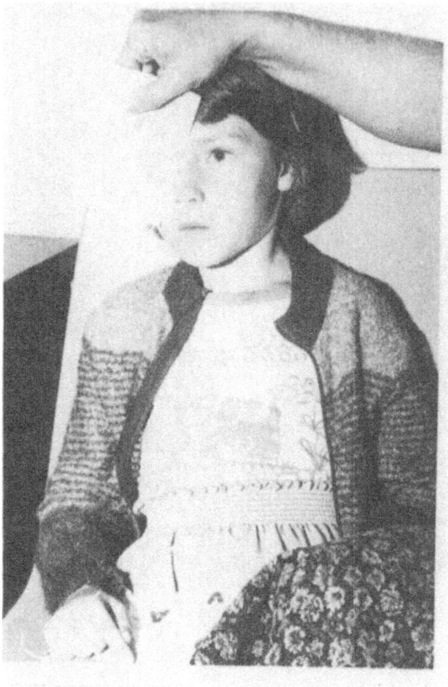

Figure 14(b) Cover test using a card (right)

Always remember that discrepancies on single-letter testing are much more significant than on a line test. It is perfectly legitimate and desirable, though often difficult, to assist a child by pointing to a letter in a normal Snellen line if this is all that is available.

References

1. Egan, D.F., Illingworth, R.S. and MacKeith, R.C. (1969). Developmental screening. 0–5 years. In Gardiner, P.,

MacKeith, R. and Smith, V. (eds.) *Aspects of Developmental and Paediatric Ophthalmology* (*Clinics in Developmental Medicine* No. 32) (London: S.I.M.P. with Heinemann Medical)

2. Sheridan, Mary D. (1969). Vision screening procedures for very young or handicapped children. In Gardiner, P., MacKeith, R. and Smith, V. (eds.) *Aspects of Developmental and Paediatric Ophthalmology* (*Clinics in Developmental Medicine* No. 32) (London: S.I.M.P. with Heinemann Medical)

3. Maclellan, A.V. and Harber, P. (1979). Mobile orthoptic service for primary screening of visual disorder in young children. *Br. Med. J.*, **1**, 994–995

4. Sheridan, Mary D. (1979). The clinical assessment of visual competence in babies and young children. In Smith, V. and Keen, J. (eds.) *Visual Handicap in Children* (*Clinics in Developmental Medicine* No. 73) (London: S.I.M.P. with Heinemann Medical)

5. Gardiner, P.A. (1970). Sheridan–Gardiner test for visual acuity. *Br. Med. J.*, **2**, 108–109

6. Gardiner, P.A. (1973). A colour vision test for young children and the handicapped. *Dev. Med. Child Neurol.*, **15**, 437–440

Chapter 4

OPTICS AND REFRACTION

CHANGES IN DIMENSION OF THE GLOBE DURING GROWTH

The analogy of the eye to a camera is useful because both are optical systems governed by optical laws. It follows that accurate vision depends on the optical system of the eye being co-ordinated during growth and ideally requires a flexibility which will focus close up as well as in the far distance. Although both the eye and the camera consist of a series of refracting surfaces focusing light on a sensitive membrane, the camera is made to specification whereas the eye develops and grows and therefore might be expected to exhibit disorders arising from disorderly growth. It is one of the more mysterious manifestations of nature, especially when we are considering a millimetre as a very influential degree of deviation, that the complex relationships of the corneal curvature, anterior chamber depth, lens surface curvatures and its thickness together with the total axial length of the eye ball usually start their postnatal existence so that normal vision is possible. Growth is so co-ordinated that postnatal developmental divergences from normality, though the biggest sources of abnormal vision, are still comparatively rare.

The term refraction is not easy for everyone to understand, but some idea of its meaning is essential for knowing how the eye functions. Refraction is the power of a transparent structure to bend light rays.

This power depends largely on the curvatures of the surfaces and in a complex system like the eye also on the distances of the surfaces from each other. Each surface is a component in the total refraction of the eye. With constant curvature of the anterior part of the eye it is the length of the anteroposterior axis which determines whether the eye is long sighted or short sighted (Figure 15). This is probably the most important single dimension, but cannot be considered in isolation. In clinical practice it is the total refraction of the eye which is the quantity

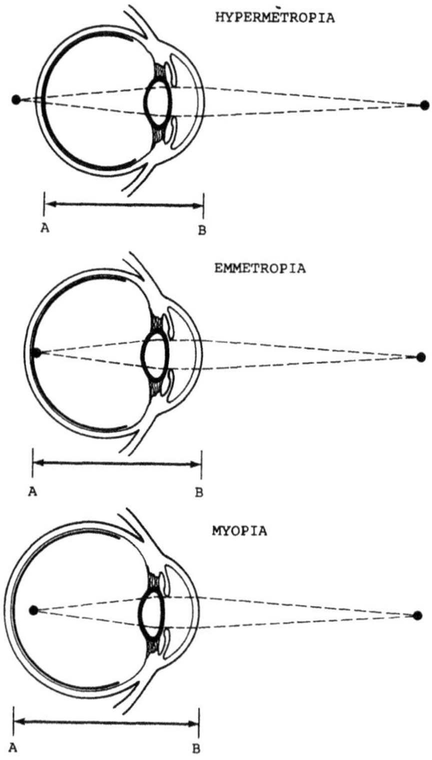

Figure 15 Dimensions determining long and short sight. This illustrates that the anteroposterior axis (A–B) is greater in myopia than in hypermetropia

determining hypermetropia, myopia or astigmatism. Long sight is synonymous with hypermetropia and short sight with myopia. In healthy eyes the visual defect arising from virtually any refraction anomaly can be compensated for by lenses, whether spectacle or contact. The estimation of the lens necessary is arrived at clinically by the process of retinoscopy. This is termed performing a refraction or refracting the eye. It is an essential basic procedure in all cases of abnormal sight where the media are transparent and particularly so in young children because if the refraction is abnormal it is certain that there is a visual defect and that without glasses it will remain so.

One important influence on the outcome is obviously the state of the infant's sight at birth. Though normal relationships are the rule some are born highly hypermetropic and some highly myopic, many with minor variations. The two extremes come to light earlier in life owing to their causing impaired vision, but even so few are noticed at birth without special testing, and studies of refractive changes during growth seldom include babies. Those that do are open to suspicion on the grounds of technical difficulties in estimation. Therefore, even the normal changes in refraction in infancy, if any, are still uncertain. High myopia in infants is unlikely to change significantly in contradistinction to the acquired myopia of middle childhood. The same lack of change applies to most cases of infantile high hypermetropia, but there is no such thing as acquired high hypermetropia. The evidence may be biased, as most hypermetropia studied from infancy is associated with squints. Refractive evidence that is not based on full cycloplegia is likely to be inaccurate and for this reason alone many reports of infant refraction of whole populations are of little value.

Newer techniques, including ultrasonography and photographic measures, hold out hopes of increasing knowledge, but one of the biggest limiting factors even then is the difficulty of knowing precisely which axis is being measured and its relation to visual fixation.

Theoretically, the growth of the eyeball with lengthening of its anteroposterior axis by 6 mm (normally) would lead to myopia of about 15 dioptres (see below), but the compensating alterations of corneal and lens curvatures prevent this. Most of this growth occurs in the early years of life, whereas the commonest age span in which failure to co-ordinate occurs in those who acquire myopia is between 7 and 14 years.

A dioptre (D) is defined as the reciprocal of the focal length expressed in metres and is the numerical expression of the amount a given lens can alter the path of the rays passing through it.

Positive values = convex lenses for hypermetropia.

Negative values = concave lenses for myopia.

These are spherical lenses. Lenses for astigmatism are cylindrical and this is indicated in a prescription by $\pm x$ D *cyl*. The conclusion is that the co-ordination of growth of the eye is normally very strict. It is debatable whether acquired myopia in later childhood is primarily anything to do with growth, whether of the eye or its owner. This is a topic which requires separate consideration together with a description of other refractive anomalies.

There is a welter of data, 'many contradictory, on these optical dimensions, but one repeated finding is that the female cornea is more curved than the male. Not only is the female cornea on average more curved than the male, but she has a shorter eye than he does. It follows that in studying populations the sex distribution is most important, seeing that these are powerful factors in the make-up of the total refraction.

Sorsby[2] gives a reliable though possibly limited picture of certain of these changes. He reports that between the age of 3 and 15 years there is a reduction in total refraction of 1.4 D and 2.3 D in boys and girls respectively.

These figures take no account of race and social class, both of which will affect the figures in some way. These mean figures, however, represent wide variations in the various components in individuals which still result in normal acuity.

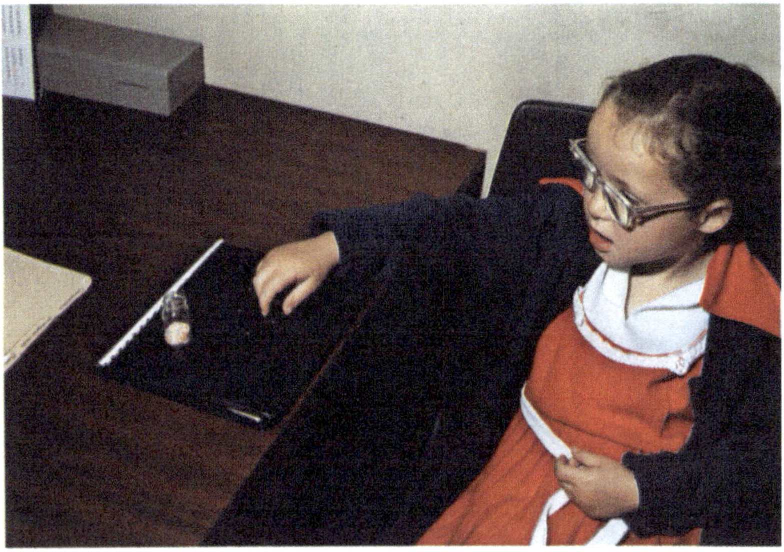

Figure 6 Testing near vision with Hundreds and Thousands

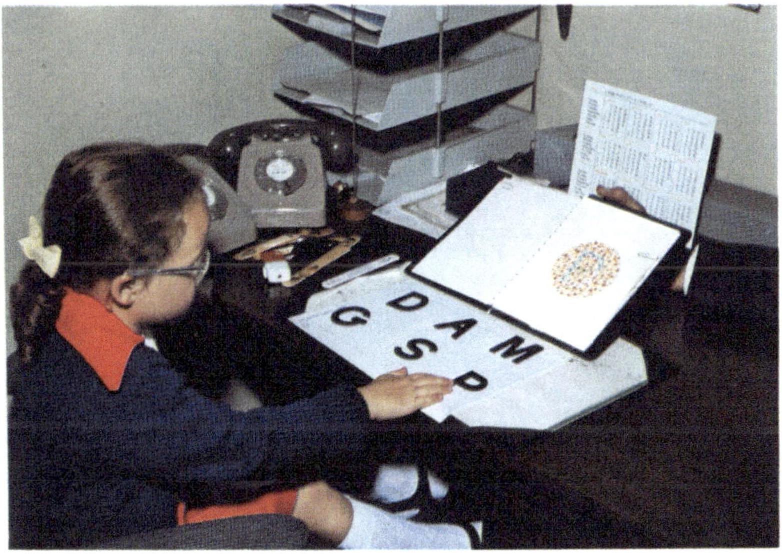

Figure 13 Colour-vision matching test

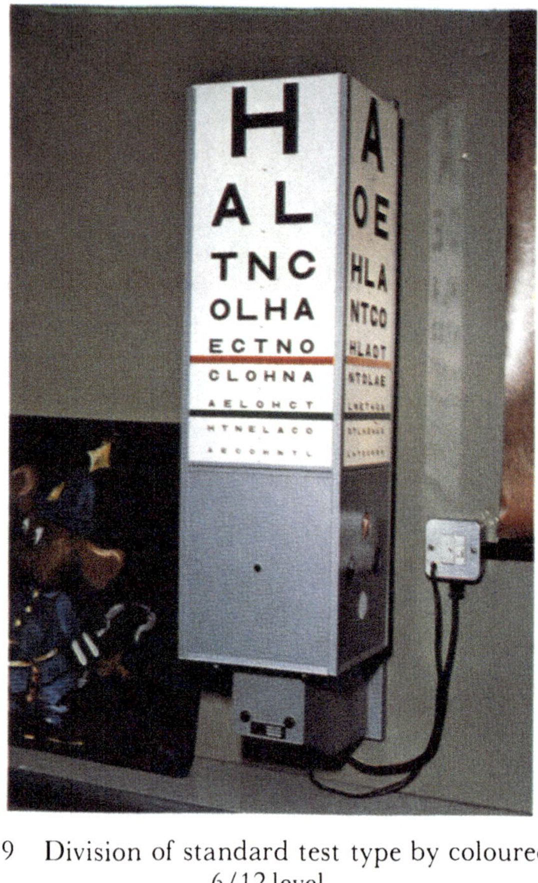

Figure 19 Division of standard test type by coloured line at 6/12 level

Over the age of 10 years he found that hypermetropes show less axial elongation than emmetropes, who in turn change less than myopes. The average lens power declined by some 1.5 D between 3 and 13, which is a very small amount. Such evidence as there is suggests the axial length of the eye to be about 18 mm in infants and 23 mm when aged 3 years so that in this period one might expect more changes in total refraction to occur than in the ensuing 10 years, when the change in length is only one-fifth of this amount spread over such a long period. There is no reliable evidence that there are larger changes in refraction in the first 3 years than at later ages in childhood.

THE VISUAL EFFECTS OF REFRACTIVE ANOMALIES

The optical system of the eye demands that a focused image be produced on the retina if accurate vision is to be obtained. If one accepts this as the essential point of the system the refractive power of the eye may be found to be correctly co-ordinated, as it is in most, or it may be inadequately adjusted in three different ways. Rays may be focused in front of or behind the retina. These constitute myopia and hypermetropic spherical errors respectively. The third anomaly is when the horizontal and vertical axes have different powers, thus producing the cylindrical effect known as astigmatism. Relative to the retina this asymmetrical effect can give a focused image behind or in front of the retina in one axis and the opposite in the other axis, including of course many other instances where one focused axis is on the retina. The general effect of astigmatism in terms of vision is somewhat similar to the distorting mirrors in funfairs (Figure 16).

None of these refractive anomalies should be called diseases; all are maladjustments of the optical measurements of the eye. Clinical experience supports the opinion that with the exception of the special case of acquired myopia all are congenital conditions or possibly may arise in early infancy. Thereafter

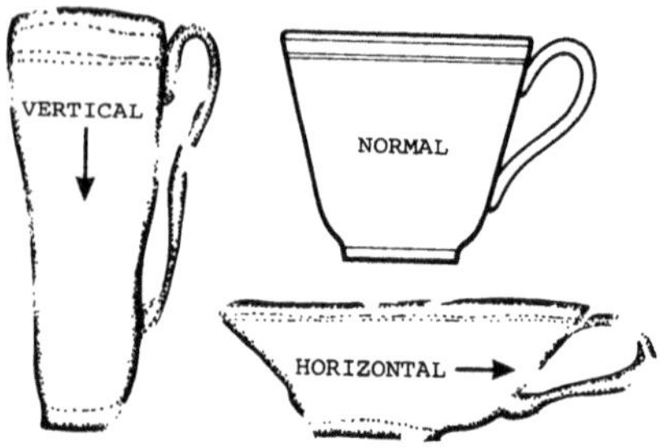

Figure 16 Distortion caused by astigmatic refraction. The normal cup is seen elongated and blurred according to the axis of the astigmatism

there appears to be little change in some 90% of children throughout their growing period and beyond.

Failure to perform a refraction in infancy has condemned many a child to years of indifferent acuity or even to a lifetime of poorer vision than might have been developed. It is impossible to overcome significant degrees of refractive anomaly by will power, exercises or even practice since nearly all these anomalies depend on physical quantities of a structural kind similar to, for example, the shape of the nose or the size and curve of a fingernail. Normal sight depends on such curvatures in the eye and on its total dimensions being related in exactly the correct amount; more depends on these minute physical measurements for correct function in the eye than anywhere else in the body.

Refraction is the objective measurement on which the power of any glasses prescribed is based. It requires a certain amount of practice to estimate the basic refraction. The need for ophthalmologists and opticians arises because it requires a great deal of practice and experience to interpret the figures arrived at in terms of the need for glasses, or of the effect of a given anomaly of refraction on eyesight, especially in anyone who cannot communicate freely. Nearly all children under the age of 10 have some such problem of communication in an eye test including a refraction and infants of course can give no answers. This is not to be wondered at, since many adults regard such tests as an ordeal and find it difficult to answer the questions they are asked.

Nearly everyone knows that 'eye testing' comprises a quite intricate question and answer programme and it often baffles the adult how this can be replaced in infants and children. The answer is that the figures provided by accurate refraction supply enough information for a prescription and that the question and answer programme is a refinement to arrive at the best glasses rather than just useful glasses.

Refraction in young children is in fact a more essential procedure than in adults, especially if no reliable evidence of visual acuity can be obtained, because it tells the examiner for sure whether a given eye has the potentiality of good vision. If the refraction is normal then the presumption is that acuity is also. The acuity *must* be lower than normal in the presence of a refractive anomaly. This information is particularly desirable in infants and young children coming from families with known visual defects which arose early in life. Useful glasses can be prescribed without any further information so that the child from then on is provided with a normal optical system enabling him to see the world more clearly, though it may take time (see adaptation, amblyopia, p. 82) for this improvement to become manifest.

In theory no infant is too young for spectacles, but the practical difficulties of wear and fitting are an obstacle. Contact lenses are sometimes a satisfactory substitute, but require continuous supervision and dedication beyond the powers of most parents, and intermittent wear is unlikely to be of much benefit.

Accommodation

The description of the value of refraction and its exercise has omitted one major developmental difference between adults and children which affects the results to a great degree, namely the faculty of accommodation. This is more powerful in children and is highly active. Accommodation affects visual acuity, especially for near vision, and when active is a component in refraction. It is also a major factor in producing squints.

It often puzzles adults why children's refraction is carried out with drops. The reason is that paralysing the accommodation (cycloplegia) is the only certain way in children and infants of estimating how much of the total refraction is made up of the static optical structural system, which is a rigid anatomical quantity, and how much it is influenced by the accommodative effect, which is functional, dynamic and variable. Hypermetropes have to exercise an amount of accommodation for distance vision as well as for near. As they age, though often not until adulthood, even those who have managed without glasses will need them due to failing accommodation, mainly for near vision but increasingly for distance. Refraction under cycloplegia shows the true degree of hypermetropia and is a reliable guide to the amount of accommodative effort required. Consequently the most appropriate strength of glasses can be ordered.

Accommodation in hypermetropes and in normal eyes serves a useful purpose, but in myopia of any severity it is not needed. It can still be exercised even to such an extent that the amount of myopia present can be greatly overestimated. Glasses may be ordered in some cases quite unnecessarily, in others much stronger than is truly required. Secondary conditioning to these glasses can occur and lead to apparent progression of a condition which was never there in the first place. Therefore, in the young myope also cycloplegia is necessary to eliminate the effects of accommodation at the time of refraction. In the long term accommodation in most myopes tends to weaken owing to its uselessness, since all myopes can read close to their eyes without glasses and without exercising accommodation (Table 1).

The non-specialist and the public are needlessly worried by

the presence of an astigmatic refraction. In fact neglected myopia and hypermetropia are as often the cause of a permanent visual defect which cannot be remedied as is astigmatism. Secondary changes in myopia later in life, unrelated to the use or abuse of glasses, sometimes even cause blindness – which never results either from hypermetropia or astigmatism. *Per se* none result in significant visual handicap if properly handled in the early years.

These conditions in infancy and early childhood are mostly dealt with by ophthalmologists (or should be) because of their potentiality for causing serious visual handicap, but anyone concerned with developmental medicine should have enough knowledge to be able to monitor how a child's problems are being attended to and be able to judge the value of any programme which appears to lie ahead of the child. In particular he should be able to interpret for the patient the language of the ophthalmologist or optician.

POPULAR MISCONCEPTIONS

Common terms which mislead are often used and the following should be avoided, however hallowed by tradition, because of their implication rather than the terms themselves:

(1) Eyestrain.
(2) Weak eyes or sight.

An example of popular misconceptions was chanced on in a television interview. A well-educated newscaster asked her portrait painter whether he had difficulty in painting her eyes correctly as she had an astigmatism. She is not alone in thinking that an astigmatism is something visible to the outsider, but ophthalmologists have to use retinoscopy to detect it even in its grossest forms.

Attitudes to beware of rest on all sorts of statements, allegedly from professionals, such as 'You will go blind if you wear the wrong glasses too often or the right glasses too seldom'; 'His sight is much worse because his glasses are becoming stronger and stronger'. This is seldom true because the common cause in children of 'increasing strength' of glasses is myopia, which affects distance acuity only. It is of the utmost reassurance to myopes and their parents to demonstrate how their near vision is excellent and unchanging. Both hypermetropia and astigmatism, if of a high order, cause more handicap because both near and distance vision are defective. A compensating factor is that neither hypermetropes nor astigmats change very much. This stability is a happy but rather illusory benefit as compared with sometimes frequent changes in young myopes.

PERMANENT DISABILITY

Permanent changes which cannot be helped by glasses arise in two ways, leading to permanent visual defect. A refractive disorder in existence from birth produces an inaccurate image on the retina. The persistence of this over the early years of life, i.e. during the years when visual development is most active, leads to adaptation to the defect, part of which may include a cortical or perceptive ignorance of the nature of clarity. This can be so severe that the potential ability to see clearly is obliterated in some and in others is limited. In both cases this results in only a limited appreciation of the clear image presented by glasses and therefore a permanent visual defect is created by the failure to initiate treatment early enough in life (but see anisometropia).

This limitation is one form of amblyopia and is a possibility common to all marked refractive anomalies, though more so in high hypermetropia or astigmatism than in myopia. This may be because the cortex receives clear images in myopia of near objects, whereas in the others both near and distance vision are affected. These effects are common in children whose eyes have unequal refraction (anisometropia). A unilateral congenital myope will often see well with a glass for the affected eye, though it may take time for the acuity to develop fully, even if a year or two has gone by before discovery of the defect. A unilateral hypermetrope or astigmat in similar circumstances is much less likely to see well and often no better with a glass. This can be tackled by occluding the good eye at the cost of blurring the child's vision (see occlusion, p. 51). If this treatment works, i.e. the acuity with glasses is improved, the condition often reverts when the occlusion is removed. Something permanent is achieved, however, because normal or improved cortical patterns, even if they are not used, remain as a potential skill which can be redeveloped if the better eye fails later in life.

What may seem a pointless exercise to parents or a failure of treatment is in a way effecting an insurance policy. Occlusion has its dangers and is discussed more fully in the section on squints. Anisometropia is more commonly found in squinting children than in children with straight eyes and is to some extent a stumbling block to effective treatment of the squint.

A much rarer late result of failure to treat a bilateral refractive disorder at an early age or in the case of acquired myopia at an early stage is that of 'non-tolerance'. This is the inability to tolerate clear vision when it is provided. It is more common in myopes though not unknown in hypermetropes. It is a condition of later childhood because by definition a threshold of toleration has already been achieved, which would not be the case in the adaptable stage of early infancy. Myopia as a refractive anomaly is only similar to astigmatism and hypermetropia in that there is a congenital form. Unlike astigmatism and hypermetropia, however, the common form of myopia is acquired, whereas acquired hypermetropia is unknown, except pathologically, though small increases sometimes occur. Astigmatism is acquired to any great degree only in rare pathological conditions.

SPECIAL FEATURES OF MYOPIA[1]

Myopia differs from hypermetropia and astigmatism not only because in most cases it is acquired, but also because it tends to increase in amount intermittently from the time of its first appearance. There is little evidence that it appears in this form before the age of 5 years.

It also differs from the other forms of refractive anomaly in being strongly associated later on in life with pathological changes in the retina, leading to serious and permanent visual loss. These changes may cause detachment of the retina if they are in its periphery. When they are in the centre of the retina they cause distortion of print or blind spots in the central field. Both these can cause serious visual handicap. Their impact is enhanced because they commonly appear at ages when active life is at its height. They are very rare as developmental processes but appear to be their consequence. These changes occur in only a small proportion of myopes, but myopia is such a common condition that they become major items in the causes of visual handicap and blindness in Western cultures.

Table 1 Acuity and accommodation in refractive anomalies

Anomaly	*Accommodation required*		*Effect on visual acuity*	
	Near	*Distance*	*Near*	*Distance*
High hypermetropia	++	+	Impaired	Impaired
Moderate hypermetropia	+	±	Impaired	Normal
Astigmatism	+*	Nil†	Impaired	Impaired
Myopia	±	Nil	Normal	Impaired

*Unless combined with myopia. †Unless combined with hypermetropia.

Table 1 shows that glasses may be needed for all these conditions, though mostly for distance vision in myopes and, for visual defects, more often constantly in the higher degrees of hypermetropia and astigmatism. Clinically, near-vision defects are not noticeably a handicap in young children, but may become so when a great deal of reading of smaller print becomes necessary in later childhood.

There is one other consideration. The scheme suggests that myopes do not require glasses for near vision. There are two schools of thought about this and no strong evidence in favour of either.

Optically correct glasses compensate for the optical defects present. Therefore, if glasses are worn by myopes for near vision the amount of accommodation required becomes normal and the situation is more akin to usual physiological mechanisms than to allow a child to grow up neglecting a normal faculty.

Others believe that accommodation causes myopia or its progress. These practitioners not only order glasses but order bifocal glasses to abolish the use of any accommodation whatever. The rationale for this is unclear because all normal children, and hypermetropes even more, do exercise their accommodation. The argument that accommodation causes myopia would logically lead us to expect that those who use it the most, i.e. hypermetropes, would be the most likely to alter their refraction towards myopia. In fact they are the most stable throughout development.

There is one further minor pragmatic argument on tolerance. If a myopic child never wears glasses for near vision, he is not only performing an unphysiological act, but also adapting himself so that it becomes difficult or impossible to read with glasses. He is therefore likely to be handicapped in later years because of the necessity to remove his glasses for all near work or to rely on bifocal glasses, and is therefore less versatile in situations where rapid changes of focus are required.

Even more minor reasons for wearing glasses almost constantly are that they can always be found and are less likely to be damaged. Most middle-aged and older persons know the force of this argument.

THE ROLE OF GLASSES IN REFRACTIVE ANOMALIES

Glasses are to be recommended to enable a child to see what he cannot see without them. Except in the special case of squints there is no virtue of any kind in older children wearing glasses which do not improve their acuity either for near or distance vision and all except the most docile will reject them. There is no convincing evidence in older children that glasses prevent changes for the worse in myopia and the same applies to contact lenses, though the changes required of contact lenses are fewer than of spectacle lenses for a given increase in myopia, which gives spurious evidence that changes are not occurring so rapidly. This is for the optical reason that they are worn nearer the eye.

There is also no convincing evidence in older children that failure to wear glasses which improve acuity has any deleterious effect other than handicapping the child's activities.

In younger children (aged up to 10) their use is different because of their assistance in the development of accurate cortical interpretation of visual stimuli. Even in those children with no apparent immediate visual benefit this usually gradually occurs with use. Whether this ultimately leads to 'dependence' on glasses is irrelevant. In some cases they can and should be dispensed with and in others their use must continue. It is perfectly possible to prescribe glasses and condition young children to their use unnecessarily, even to the extent of producing an artificial defect of acuity without them. These are the basic reasons for giving children special attention in special clinics where their needs are not judged by standards in adults.

References

1. Gardiner, P.A. (1979). Epidemiology of myopia. In Smith, V. and Keen, J. (eds.) *Visual Handicap in Children* (*Clinics in Developmental Medicine* No. 73) (London: S.I.M.P. with Heinemann Medical)

2. Sorsby, A., Benjamin, J. and Sheridan, M. (1960). Refraction and its components. *MRC Special Report*

Chapter 5

SQUINTS

Squints can be caused by several pathological conditions in the eye and by general medical conditions. The commoner causes are listed below. By far the commonest squint in childhood arises at birth or in the early years and has none of these causes. Until we understand the cause of these squints fully we must look at them as a developmental problem because they arise in childhood and must be dealt with in childhood if any results other than cosmetic are to be obtained.

The following description is an attempt to put into perspective the process of treatment of the common squint and its likely results together with the visual problems incurred. The community physician, paediatrician or general practitioner is likely to be the first medical contact and will, if only intermittently, make comments or give a guiding hand so he will be helped if he has some insight into the different aspects of the condition.

USE OF THE TERM 'SQUINT'

The word squint is interpreted differently by different people. Most doctors in Britain mean the state of affairs where the two eyes are not parallel. This is, however, not quite accurate, because where the gaze is at something close to, the eyes are (or should be) convergent and a squint is not present. The best meaning is to consider a squint as being present whenever the two eyes are not looking at the same object.

This may clarify the meaning in the doctor's mind, but it

does nothing for the patient whose mother perhaps has brought him for what she thinks may be a 'lazy eye'. Or, as in one instance of an obvious squint, the mother replied in answer to 'How long has he had a squint?' that: 'He hasn't got a squint, it's his cross eye that worries me.' It is doubtful if this confusion will ever be resolved and it is particularly obstructive when family history is being recounted. Many an adult with a squint and amblyopia will deny having had a squint, but admit a lazy eye. Many others will claim to squint because they often peer through half-closed lids. This is the method whereby myopes see more clearly and is often the first sign of short sight in childhood, but has nothing to do with a squint. Yet another term used by the public is a cast.

Almost everywhere in the world, including the USA, the term strabismus is used for incorrect alignment and confusion is much less. However the normal English parent's reaction to this term is one of anxiety and she will be greatly relieved to hear it is another word for a squint.

All squints may have a pathological cause rather than merely being a state of neuromuscular inco-ordination associated with optical or visual anomalies.

THE COMMONER PATHOLOGICAL CAUSES OF SQUINT

(A) All ages

(1) Systemic infections whether viral or bacterial.
(2) Demyelinating diseases.
(3) Vascular disease.
(4) Cerebral neoplasms.
(5) Poisoning (e.g. lead).
(6) Myaesthenia gravis.
(7) Trauma (e.g. blow-out fractures of the orbit).
(8) Orbital neoplasms, inflammation, oedema (e.g. thyroid disease) and circulatory anomalies.

(9) Inflammatory disease of sinuses or ear.
(10) Any uniocular loss of vision.

(B) Children

(1) Birth trauma.
(2) Aplasia or other abnormalities of oculomotor nuclei and in general any intracerebral condition which may affect their connections such as, for instance, hydrocephalus or meningitis.
(3) Absence or poor development of extraocular muscles.
(4) Retinoblastoma (rare but lethal).
(5) Cataract.
(6) Toxoplasmosis.
(7) Rubella.
(8) Any infectious fever in childhood.

In addition there are:

(1) Emotional (usually transient).
(2) Stress (such as teething), again usually transient.
(3) Voluntary convergence, which can become permanent.

Squints are therefore a medical problem until proved otherwise. Doctors and their patients should seek further advice in all cases. All children should attend a doctor the first time ophthalmic advice is thought to be necessary. The divorce of a general practitioner's interest from visual problems is unwise at any age, but its effect on the care of infants and young children can be harmful without a comprehensive active community service charged with the supervision of visual defects.

Medical neglect or spontaneous parental action can result in fruitless and time-wasting journeying to the optician during the weeks or months when diagnosis and the initiation of treatment are most urgent. Screening for squint and developmental assessment from an early age has become much more important since general practitioners gave up their introductory role to the General Ophthalmic Service. The possible methods are outlined later.

Whether they should be undertaken by the GP or under the auspices of the community paediatrician is debatable, but without universal screening or at least particular attention to special groups, many cases with permanent impairment of visual potential will be missed and many more will have delayed recognition.

Apart from the possibility of missing a lethal condition, the danger of leaving a squint is that the child will grow into it and adapt to it rather than grow out of it.

The diagnosis of squints lies largely on the corneal light reflex (Figure 17) and the cover test, both of which are not always easy to interpret (see page 41).

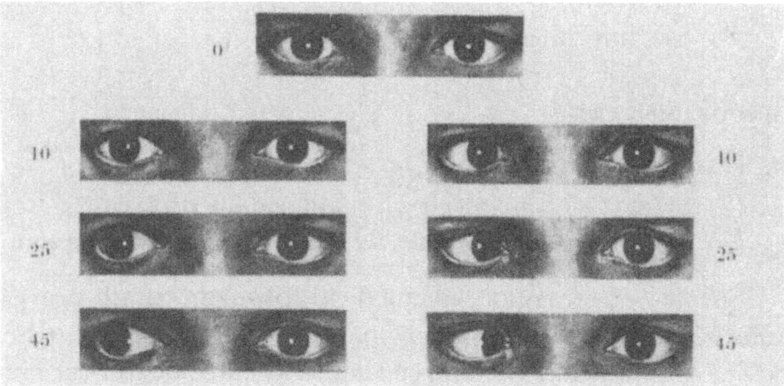

Figure 17 Corneal reflex test. The normal corneal reflex is at the top and is symmetrical. The reflexes in the left column show greatly increasing divergence of the right eye and in the right column similarly increasing convergence [from Duke Elder (1979), *System of Ophthalmology*, Vol. 5 (Henry Kimpton), by kind permission]

Many a parent will claim to have grown out of a squint without treatment, but this is seldom the truth and it should be disregarded. The reason for the statement is either that the squint was only an illusory one due to the breadth of the nose or that something like peering is being referred to.

EPICANTHUS

Epicanthus is only of importance because its presence fakes a squint, as will be seen from Figure 18. If the fold of skin is eliminated by pinching it up at the bridge of the nose the 'squint' disappears. Most mothers are convinced by the demonstration, some only reluctantly.

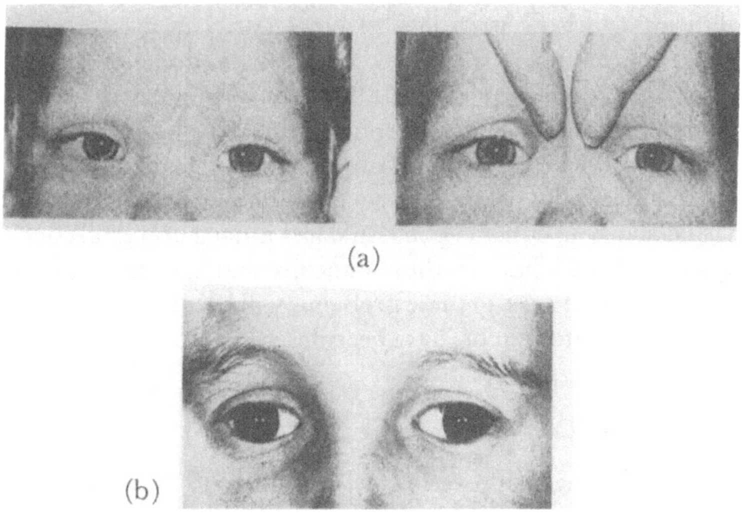

Figure 18 (a) Pseudo-convergent squint, due to a large separation of the two inner canthi-epicanthal folds, eliminated by pinching the skin over the bridge of the nose. (b) Pseudo-divergent squint, due to inward displacement of the outer canthi [from Duke Elder (1979), *System of Ophthalmology*, Vols. 5 and 6 (Henry Kimpton), by kind permission]

Parents sometimes bring photographs of themselves as infants as confirmation; but a squint cannot be diagnosed by a still photograph, however vivid or genuine the appearance may seem. Apart from the condition of epicanthus, the normal convergence to a near object may be the cause of the camera's record.

THE CONSEQUENCES OF SQUINTS

Many people think that defective binocular vision must lead to failure to appreciate depth or to diplopia, but this is not the case in squints arising in infancy or in early childhood. The young child's ability to compensate or adapt to defects overcomes any difficulties arising from lack of binocularity in his daily life. Most ophthalmologists have come across examples of outstanding skills achieved by adults with very poor or absent binocular vision. These include surgical colleagues, racing motorists, cricketers or tennis players, sometimes of top class.

An alternating squint of early onset does not result in loss of visual acuity in either eye so visual loss is not a universal consequence. If so, what are the handicaps that a squinting child suffers? The answer to these problems will become clearer once all the associated factors have been described.

SUPPRESSION

Understanding suppression is essential to understanding squints. The study of suppression supports a belief in critical stages of development and in a 'learning' factor in visual performance which is more active in early childhood, less active later and which disappears altogether by early adolescence. Though suppression has a negative effect it is a positive process.

Some general considerations apply. A normal feature of human life and consciousness is that events which occurred in early childhood are forgotten. It is arguable that this is not a lapse of memory but a suppression of what most observers would gladly know nothing about. If the general infantile unpleasantness of incontinence, vomiting, inco-ordination, immobility and frustration – all of which is punctuated by noisy distress – is hard to tolerate, it is an understandable benefit that none of it is remembered.

A degree of suppression in adults of unwanted or uninteresting sounds or of pain can occur, but usually only in exceptional circumstances. In battle minor wounds or injuries are not noticed, in long-distance running the scenery is not noticed, in rowing a race the concentration of propulsion suppresses the pain from a boil on the bottom, during intense emotion sense of time and of outside events are lost or confused. Hunger may be suppressed by excitement, fatigue is suppressed in the team performing a surgical operation and, though it is not a common experience, poets and fakirs can suppress what the common man would say was insuppressable when they partake in their particular abstraction from the world. All these are in a sense suppression by diversion by concentrating on the important event. They are not lapses of memory and are only partial.

Most of this suppression is beneficial and is contrary to the Freudian theory that all should be brought to the surface.

What is the relevance of this mechanism to visual development? It is a commonplace in medical practice to come across adults who, because of injury or disease, suffer from paralysis of one or more of the extraocular muscles. This causes double vision in those with normal binocular vision. When this persists often the only solution is to occlude one eye by some means.

This is not the position in childhood after a similar paralysis. In young children the rule is for single vision to become stabilized after quite a short time by the mechanism of suppression. For example, a child born with a paralysed external rectus muscle can be shown to have binocular vision except in the field where the defective muscle operates. As soon as an abduction in that direction occurs binocular vision switches off and confusing double images are suppressed. In older children this may not occur. Adaptation to intermittent diplopia is also possible in inconstant squints which begin before school age.

Adaptation and suppression are not the same process

because certain types of diplopia can be abolished by assuming abnormal head posture. The form of adaptation in intermittent divergent squints, for example, may not be to overcome the diplopia by making one image disappear, but by recognizing the real image rather than the unreal image. This is easier if one image is blurred.

These diplopia phenomena are so much an acceptable part of such a child's life that they are seldom reported and often are elicited only by direct questioning by the doctor. These children's mothers will say that they can't believe it and that the child is merely going along with the doctor and may even reprimand the child. This attitude is based on two assumptions. The child believes that everyone sees double occasionally because it happens to him without handicap and the parent believes that it is impossible to see double without handicap. Therefore, the child is said to be perverse not to mention it. Young children do not understand the question 'Do you see double?' and adults also will complain of double vision when they mean overlapping images. The question must be framed: 'Do you see two of things when there is only one there?' and it can be suggested that two clocks or two moons might be seen. Most children regard this as a reasonable question and those that do see double are impressed and somewhat awed or puzzled by such medical interest in an everyday occurrence.

Double vision must arise whenever the two eyes with good acuity begin to look at different objects. Suppression will soon occur in children, therefore, if confusion is not to arise in squints. In alternating squints, typically with an equal refraction and acuity in each eye, the suppression is alternate, first in one eye then the other. Equality of acuity means in effect that there is no visual benefit in using one eye rather than the other. Each eye is therefore preferred in what appears to be a haphazard way and the other's image suppressed at the same time. Equal vision in each eye, but absence of binocular vision, is the general rule in alternating squints and no diplopia occurs due to effective suppression. Suppression is so deeply rooted in many such squints of early origin that even if the eyes are straightened by surgery the two eyes still alternate in transmitting an image of an object, though this is concealed from the outsider and usually unknown to the user.

By contrast, in monocular squints where only one eye fixes and the other constantly squints, and in the absence of pathological conditions, the refraction is usually dissimilar. Even when refraction is similar the suppression which occurs constantly in the squinting eye causes a diminution of acuity in this eye. Suppression is spuriously beneficial in the very early stages of a monocular squint as it leads to relative loss of function quite rapidly in the squinting eye.

Part of the treatment in such a case is occlusion of the good eye. If this is performed too rigorously an iatrogenically caused drop in acuity occurs in the good eye in young children. This can usually be reversed if the child is young enough and the duration of the occlusion is only over a short period. Obsessional pursuit of binocular vision in older children can lead to permanent diplopia because of continual stimulus of an unfused image beyond the years when suppression is possible. The limiting age is about 8–10 years. In addition to this, suppression is so selective that in many squints in older children it can occur only at the angle of squint the child is accustomed to. If this angle is altered by surgery, by prisms or by nature, double vision or confusion arises and is often irretrievable. A squinting young woman was invited by an ophthalmologist to undergo surgery to improve her appearance. Months after the operation, though she looked normal, she was a psychiatric casualty because of her constant double vision. Surgery to restore her squint also restored her mental balance, but this cure of diplopia is difficult to achieve in such cases.

Since the faculty of suppression cannot arise *de novo* in older children and adults, squints must be treated early to obtain two eyes with useful vision. In young children there is much more potential for successful treatment than in older children and adults. Years of conditioning to faulty input, coupled with the weakening of the power to adapt whether by suppression or by other means, constitute an insurmountable obstruction and a contraindication to treatment by occlusion and other forms of stimulation in older children with long-standing squints.

Thus it is essential that eye exercises in infants and other aspects of treating squints in children are supervised by properly qualified practitioners who know the dangers and can foresee possible complications.

EARLY INVESTIGATION

The predominant task of the developmental specialist in the care of vision and in particular of squints is to see to it that the child develops the best acuity possible in each eye. Other considerations, such as binocular vision and appearance, though important, are secondary.

It now appears proved that good acuity depends on the accurate use of each retina from a very early age, so the following questions require an answer in infancy:

(1) Is either eye constantly squinting?
(2) Is there a high refractive error present bilaterally or unilaterally?
(3) Is there an opacity in the media or a disease of the retina, particularly at the posterior pole?

Any of these will interfere with the accurate use of the retina.

All three questions must be answered so that elimination of any pathological condition is required. A refraction and usually an orthoptic examination are required to eliminate elusive small-angle squints, especially in those with a family history (see Chapter 7).

The classification of squints is cumbersome, but for practical purposes there are two main questions of prognostic importance. One is whether the squint is constant or intermittent and the other is whether a constantly squinting child is preferring one eye and neglecting the other or is using each alternately.

This alternating type of squint seldom, if ever, has any effect on acuity, whereas a constantly squinting eye will always have some degree of defective acuity. The defect may be quite severe (6/60 or worse) and if left untreated will become permanent. Treatment of a developmental squint which is constantly present in one eye is an urgent matter, in terms of weeks. The later the onset the better the prognosis but only if treatment is not delayed.

Intermittent squints are less urgent. Though they may cause double vision, which children tolerate well, they are seldom associated with much visual loss. In the first 6 months of life such squints are common and can be disregarded, except in those children whose siblings or parents suffered from squints. In such cases a refraction should be carried out sometime in the first year, because in a hypermetropic child such a squint is likely to become permanent sooner or later and this outcome may be prevented.

Most intermittent convergent squints are associated with inappropriate accommodation and the angle of squint in many convergent squints of any sort is increased when the eyes are accommodating for near vision.

RELATION OF REFRACTION TO SQUINTS

The relation between hypermetropia, accommodation and squints is important. The normal visual mechanism is so arranged that to bring about binocular clear near vision there are two requirements. Firstly, the focus of each eye must be adjusted to the near point. This requires action by each ciliary muscle to increase the power of the lens. Secondly, if both eyes are to be used accurately and simultaneously they must converge to fix the object. Near vision is perfectly well achieved by one eye alone so that a monocular child is unaware of any visual disturbance or difficulty. The normal situation is that as an object comes within arm's length and closer the eyes will converge and accommodation will increase. Normally these two processes are linked and reflexly co-ordinated. The eyes of hypermetropic babies and young children who have to accommodate for distance vision may converge at the same time and become still more convergent for near. Others may be straight for distance vision and convergent (or overconvergent) for near. The amount of accommodation required can be measured by refraction under cycloplegia, which paralyses the ciliary muscle. Cycloplegic drops or ointment such as atropine and numerous substitutes achieve this. It is not enough merely to dilate the pupil, as might be done for examination; the ciliary muscle must be put out of action altogether.

Under cycloplegia it becomes difficult or impossible to read without glasses and convergence is often also abolished as it is no longer triggered off by the effect of accommodation, though the ineffectual effort sometimes increases convergence. Glasses can take the place of natural accommodation so that no action of the ciliary muscle is necessary. A true accommodative squint will disappear when appropriate glasses are worn. This will be the case regardless of the effect of the glasses on acuity. It is quite common for a squinting child to have normal unaided visual acuity, yet he may require glasses to abolish the squint. We know that the power of accommodation in childhood is much greater than in adult life and its natural weakening year by year will sometimes enable glasses to be left off eventually without bringing back the squint. In this case we can justifiably claim that glasses cured the squint, or at any rate tided over the years when the presence of a squint might have adversely affected the vision in one or other eye.

A case history of identical twin girls demonstrates the effect of treatment or its absence. Proof of identicality was supported by standard methods. These children were taken to an ophthalmologist at the age of 2 years because they were identical twins, yet only one squinted. This was verified by the ophthalmologist, who refracted the squinting twin only. She had +7.0 D of hypermetropia in each eye so that she constantly had to accommodate for distance vision as well as for near. She had a constant convergence of the right eye. Glasses did not abolish the squint and the right vision remained defective. She was given orthoptic treatment with occlusion of the left eye since the acuity in the right eye continued to reduce. She also underwent surgery. Nothing was done for the twin without a squint.

When 7 years old the treated twin saw 6/12 with her right eye with glasses and 6/6 in the left. The untreated twin was found to have unaided vision of 6/6 in the right eye and less than 6/60 in the left. Refraction showed a normal right eye but an equally hypermetropic left eye as her sister's two eyes. The vision in her left eye did not improve with glasses. Therefore, both children saw 6/6, though only out of one eye, but the girl with straight eyes had far worse vision in her hypermetropic eye than her squinting twin who had received treatment. The explanation is that refraction was performed on only one child so the unequal refraction in the girl with straight eyes was missed. She spent all her formative years neglecting one eye (though it was straight) and using her normal eye. With her normal right eye she had no need to accommodate greatly, either for near or distance vision, therefore there was no stimulus to converge abnormally at any distance and the squint mechanism was not switched on. The cost to her was that she had one permanently visually defective eye which did not respond to glasses. Neither child had binocular depth perception. At 7 this situation is likely to persist for life.

It must be extremely rare, if not unique, for identical twins to present with such peculiar refraction; and since they manifested two conditions commonly associated with squints, namely anisometropia in one child and hypermetropia in the other, it is a fair hypothesis that accommodation can precipitate constant squints as well as intermittent squints.

The practical lesson to be learnt is that early refraction of all siblings of squints should be carried out under cycloplegia. This can be safely neglected only if a normal acuity has been convincingly established for each eye. Early refraction of the siblings of any child with a marked refractive anomaly is also desirable[1].

It is still not the universal custom to refract infants, unless they are squinting, so the paediatrician would be wise to question any ophthalmic report where this is not mentioned.

Another lesson to be learnt from this history is the need for screening and, as a corollary, effective follow-up. Defection is extremely common amongst parents of young children and is often not allowed for in hospital systems of organizing attendances. The second twin in this case ought not to have reached 7 years old without having her amblyopic eye discovered. She had had an acuity screening at 6 years old and stated that she dodged the occlusion (a self-held wooden spoon), thus using her good eye twice (see examination and screening).

CONTINUING TREATMENT AND SUPERVISION

A cautionary note must be sounded. Presenting glasses to a young child is not enough. He must wear them, and even this is unlikely, except for myopes, to produce an enhanced visual acuity immediately, especially where high-power lenses are necessary or if the anomaly is unilateral. Children are sensible and resent being responsible for an appliance which encumbers them and gives no subjective benefit. The management of this problem can be very difficult.

In squinting children with unilateral high-refractive disorders and therefore with some degree of amblyopia even constant wear will seldom produce an improvement without occlusion and the child will find himself saddled not only with glasses, but a patch over his good eye. Few children take kindly to this sort of sensory crippling so that it becomes essential to keep a close watch on progress and to give constant support to the parents. Large numbers default because of the initial difficulties. Although opinions differ, many ophthalmologists advise only a relatively short period of total occlusion if no improvement is signalled. When it does occur the top limit may often not reach 6/6, so treatment may have to be abandoned relatively early. Surgery should be undertaken at this moment of peak visual performance. The level reached may be precarious and short lived so that when a visual result needs to be consolidated by surgery there is no time to be lost.

This complete and often long programme needs great care, timing and interest – hence the value of the orthoptist in the ophthalmological team. Doctors are often puzzled by the abandonment of treatment, leaving a child with an amblyopic eye (perhaps with very poor vision) and without glasses. In older treated children this is because no further improvement will occur or because suppression is so intense that glasses are useless. It is unfair to ask these children to undergo more ophthalmic investigations which it is known may lead to the prescription of yet another pair of useless glasses. There may of course be special circumstances, but usually it can be established whether a programme of medical and orthoptic work has been conscientiously devised and carried out. A useful test in older children who are those most at risk of useless treatment (around and after the age of 10) is the pinhole test. Visual improvement using the pinhole might suggest further ophthalmic advice if there has been a lapse of a year or more without treatment. Absence of a response by a competent older child usually means incurable amblyopia. Care must be taken to establish that such an eye had for years been a poor performer. A new pathological development may be overlooked unless this is done.

Surgery is performed for two main reasons. Firstly, because unless the visual axis is corrected the old defects will return; and secondly, even if no visual benefit is likely to result, the psychological disadvantage of possessing a squinting eye is quite serious, particularly in older children. The younger the age the more urgent surgery is if a visual effect is desired, and it is still too common for squints to be on waiting lists for months or years. This is wasting irretrievable formative periods, perhaps causing permanent deleterious effects.

Some believe that surgery is done mainly to achieve binocularity and that failure to become binocular is a disadvantage. This is not a drawback of any importance in daily living in young children either at the time (if of early onset) or later in their lives. Other people, particularly mothers, worry only for cosmetic reasons so that small-angle squints tend to be neglected and the case for surgery is misunderstood. In this case some preventable visual loss may be a consequence of failure to operate at the optimum moment.

Surgery cannot now be considered a major hazard or intolerable as practised in modern hospitals on a healthy child. There is a move to treat these children as day patients, since the only risk is of anaesthetic complications. The days when both eyes were bandaged and the child was admitted without his mother have gone. Only in cases of special vulnerability is a stay in hospital mandatory.

We should think about how children feel themselves. Normal children become completely aware of their disability, which colours their personalities and activities. One 8-year-old child burst into tears when he was told he would have his name put on the waiting list for surgery. This was not from fear of the operation, but from disappointment, because being a gypsy this was the fourth time his name had been entered and he had never stayed long enough in one place to come to the top of the list.

The intensity of self-conscious feeling is seldom expressed. For example, a blind girl of 16 asked to have both eyes removed for cosmetic reasons. This thought must cross many of these children's minds, but not all, so it is extremely easy to offer unprompted advice and suggest to others, who are quite happy, that their appearance is unpleasant.

Other forms of squints, i.e. divergent or vertical, occur without known pathology, but the principles of handling the problem are the same. Firstly, to diagnose early and treat suitable cases as soon as the diagnosis is made. Secondly, to aim at improving acuity where it is defective. Thirdly, to give the child straight eyes. Binocular depth perception will be added to these aims as progress is made.

The nature of the untreated disability suffered by a squinting child is now clearer. He has a much higher risk of having only one useful eye for the rest of his life. He will develop fears – whether expressed or not – about the preservation of good sight in his only useful eye, which will affect his conduct and attitude to life. He will suffer from being an obvious target for taunts from his fellows and later will come feelings of inadequacy from being unable to look the world and its inhabitants straight in the eye. This will affect his attitude to potential employment and marriage prospects. Though most of these feelings are common to all humanity the treatment of a preventable handicap of this nature should be a welcome medical responsibility, since so much can be done to relieve it if the task is undertaken early in life.

THE ORTHOPTIST AND SQUINTS

The potential role of the orthoptist has already been referred to when discussing visual screening of infants (p. 37). Historically, however, this is a by-product of her original function.

Early in the century it was recognized by ophthalmologists that binocular depth perception demanded straight eyes, and orthoptic techniques of training were developed which aimed at achieving binocularity without surgery or using it only as an adjuvant. There was once optimism that these eye exercises, analogous to the activities of physiotherapists in the realms of general muscular co-ordination and correction of malfunction, would become a major weapon in improving and perfecting binocular vision. These exercises have no relationship to the much advertised quackery which claims to provide better sight without glasses.

As time went by it became clear that orthoptics stood no chance of rectifying long-established defects which were founded on events in early childhood, because they had been conditioned and consolidated during the formative sensitive years of adaptation and of the development of visual potential. Earlier diagnosis became the cry and still is, so that at present the bulk of an orthoptist's work is with infants and young children and actual treatment of older children over the age of, say, 8 forms a minor part, especially in relation to improvement of binocular vision, which by this age has become more or less fixed. There is, however, a group of older children where good or precarious binocular vision breaks down, either with symptoms of double vision (which seldom occurs in younger children and is well tolerated) or of blurring and lachrymation, often described as strain with near vision.

Symptoms of this syndrome of ocular muscle imbalance can occur at any age after, say, 10. One variety of it is difficulty or insufficiency of convergence. The absence of symptoms in younger children when this condition is present and its comparative rarity amongst them is another indication of the different mechanisms at work in early childhood compared with later on in life. This is perhaps the main group with whom an orthoptist practises what was originally hoped to be her role of successful treatment.

This movement towards earlier and earlier diagnosis, coupled with the knowledge that normal binocular depth perception is only likely to be achieved in a few children with squints, has led to a change of emphasis in the orthoptist's role. She is now expected to take far more interest in young babies and, owing to the rapid changes in acuity which can take place in young children without their being noticeable to the inexpert, she has become well versed in methods of testing for acuity as well as for the presence or absence of a squint. She can monitor the effect of glasses and of occlusion which still form the mainstay of non-surgical treatment. Frequent testing, perhaps weekly at times, occupies many hours of work and one consequence will be discussed in the chapter on essential services. It was never expected that the orthoptist would develop this expertise and perhaps become a key figure in screening babies and infants for visual disorders yet this seems a possibility for the future.

Acuity and squinting angles can change rapidly at any time in the first 5 years, so repeated visits over a long period are necessary and good personal rapport between the orthoptist and the mother and child is essential.

INFORMING PARENTS

Parents fall roughly into three classes. Firstly, those who have or have had genuine squints themselves and know first hand what they experienced a generation ago. They also remember what they think they were told about blindness or useless vision in one eye. They have good memories of the cycloplegic ointment, usually because of the consequent week-long difficulty with reading. Their recall is often partial, misleading and of obsolete procedures.

A second group know a lot from hearsay and much of this has to be sorted out by discussion.

The third group know nothing and by temperament are often either very worried or very casual.

The commonest question asks whether the child will need glasses or not and if so for how long they will be necessary. Many will say they would prefer the operation to glasses, but fewer than before positively refuse operation. These options are not possible to meet. All squints require a balanced programme embracing the possibility of orthoptic treatment, glasses and surgery. Totally ignorant parents should be told this and knowledgeable parents told that patterns of treatment change in a generation. For example, no child has both eyes bandaged postoperatively, which used to be the rule, and stay in hospital is short compared with the week or two common in the past. A second operation must always be mentioned as a possibility in a planned programme. Parents of infants also need to be told that the programme is likely to extend over years before the final effect on the angle of squint, the visual acuity and the need for glasses is known. They should not be encouraged to think that appearance is all that counts, which is so often at the back of their minds when they express anxiety about glasses and surgery.

Reference

1. Ingram, R.M. (1977). Refraction as a basis for screening children for squint and amblyopia. *Br. J. Ophthalmol.*, **61**, 8–15

Chapter 6

OPHTHALMIC SERVICES FOR CHILDREN

It was noticed in the early twentieth century that many adults with grave congenital or developmental defects of vision had never received any advice about their eyesight. The school ophthalmic service was set up to screen children and consequently to offer ophthalmic advice to those whose sight was defective. These clinics were staffed by ophthalmologists under contract to the local authority and provided an alternative to obtaining advice for a fee from an optician or a private ophthalmologist. The remaining choice was a visit to hospital armed with a GP's letter, which was usually only granted in cases which were obviously pathological.

With the introduction of the National Health Service 'free' sight testing became general so the thriving school eye service lost one of its attractions. More recently a shortage of ophthalmologists has made it more difficult to staff these clinics and the recent abolition of the obligation for the GP to see a child before he obtains his first eye test has led to an increase in the number of babies and children being taken to the nearest optician for primary eye care. Whatever advice is given there it can hardly be called a system and places a responsibility on the optical profession, which will be unable to meet the need comprehensively.

The absence of systematic primary eye care places a premium on parental diagnosis or suspicion rather than proper visual screening of the infant population and is very inefficient. In older children it provides only a haphazard coverage where the casual and defaulting parent does nothing for her child, whereas the over-anxious parent with a child with headaches or merely under suspicion will make frequent visits to an optician (possibly more than one) until something is done. There are just as many parents who are glad to see their child given glasses as a form of treatment as there are parents who are sceptical about the necessity for them. It is easy for medical opinion to be delayed until the efficacy of any treatment to be advised is prejudiced. Delay in the case of young children may alter the prognosis adversely. In older children the fact that so many do not wear glasses which have been prescribed for them[1] indicates the wastefulness caused by a screening programme without informed clinical follow-up.

Ideally every child should have had a visual screening test before the age of 4. It is most important that certain groups of children should have an earlier competent visual assessment (see screening schedule; Table 2, p. 102)[2]. Groups requiring early strict visual assessment and refraction in the absence of positive findings include all those children with:

(1) A family history of squints, lazy eyes or cross eyes, and their siblings.
(2) A family history of high refractive anomalies originating in infancy.
(3) Premature birth or a birth weight of under 2.2 kg.
(4) Mental or physical retardation[3-6].
(5) Brain damage.
(6) Deafness.
(7) Marked behavioural disorders.

These groups should all have had definitive statements about their vision by 2 years old at the latest. There is no need for special follow-up once their acuity in each eye has been established as normal.

It is too much to hope that the parents of these children will take the initiative, so it must come from the medical services.

The hospital service has never included primary screening amongst its activities and though in theory the GP could, his training is such that he is not competent to do so without specializing to some degree. Few vocational training courses for GPs do more than pay lip service to developmental problems of vision and many ignore visual problems as a category for study.

Most of these groups need special attention because of the increased prevalence of visual defects amongst them and the difficulty of noticing these by casual observation. The deaf are included because of the increased value to them of excellent sight at all distances so that they can make a proper appreciation of their environment. One aspect of this is the benefit to them of lip reading which depends entirely on sight.

The community health services must therefore set up screening procedures, directing special attention to the groups of children of high risk or special needs, properly documenting them and taking notice of the risks to siblings. Recall must be provided for those who are not clear of minor doubts and easy reference to specialists for those with major doubts. The necessary primary tests can be performed by trained community doctors, trained health visitors, school nurses or by orthoptists[7–9]. Liaison with local paediatric and assessment clinics is desirable.

This deals with the screening side of the service, but it is more difficult to construct a suitable system of diagnosis and treatment. Logically the school eye clinics should be extended to cover an earlier age group, but these are often in difficulties with staffing levels.

Local communities need to look at the state of the services in their area and attempt to devise one for themselves, as there is little chance of central or regional authorities modifying their priorities or breaking away from the adult-orientated practices which they have upheld for so long.

Since a large part of the diagnostic work includes refraction it would be a progressive step if local medical authorities could look to opticians to perform sessional duties, rather as their forebears called in ophthalmologists to care for the neglected eyesight of the child population.

Children would be seen first by an ophthalmologist, who would send all those he wished to have refracted to the optician. The optician and the referring ophthalmologist would confer on the possible need for glasses, further follow-up or other treatment. Most of these children could then be left to the optician for recall and supervision according to the demands of the case as assessed by the ophthalmologist. Some would be referred to hospital by the ophthalmologist and some to the local orthoptic clinic. It would be advantageous if such a service dovetailed with the hospital service rather than acted as a rival, and common appointments of staff should be favoured. A step forward would be the appointment of a local consultant who would take an interest in such community preventive measures outside hospital as part of his duties. This would include the giving of advice to schools for the handicapped in the locality whether for visually, physically or mentally handicapped, all of which often find it difficult to cater for visual problems.

FOR AND AGAINST SCREENING FOR VISUAL DEFECTS

The value of screening might appear to be incontrovertible, but many doctors' minds have become confused by the amount of effort or expertise used for what often turn out to be poor returns. This seems to apply to such investigations as measuring the blood pressure in a population with a view to preventing or forecasting cardiovascular disease in individuals. Though some correlation is obviously found at the higher values, virtually all of these would be known anyway.

Similarly, screening populations for glaucoma fails to show much predictive value – less than a knowledge of the family history. These failures have cast doubt on wholesale screening, but the argument is far from definitive. If, for instance, family history is of predictive value then this is where the screening should be applied to a whole population, and the criticism is not of the principle but of the method. When pulmonary tuberculosis was widespread, mass radiography was a measure which detected the disease at an earlier stage than established clinical tests and for that reason was welcome, but on the debit side had to be entered the number of false-positives, together with the anxiety caused by the doubtfully positive leading to supervision and recall. As the prevalence of the disease declined mass radiography became more and more expensive in terms of cases detected, and yet another factor loomed up – the possible danger of repeated exposure to X-rays.

All these considerations must enter the equation which is drawn up before a screening programme is approved. In ophthalmic work there is no alternative to screening the whole population if every defective eye is to be found. Without a screening programme of some kind in early childhood many squints affecting acuity in one eye at least will be missed at the most favourable time for remedial measures and a considerable proportion of visual defects of a handicapping nature will be overlooked to the detriment of the general progress of the young child. In view of the acquired nature of some visual defects – notably myopia in later childhood – screening once, in early childhood, is not enough. This is not to say that universal screening is practicable.

A SCREENING PROGRAMME

Jan, Freeman and Scott[10] reported that at the end of a 35-year period better surveillance and health education led to all suspected congenitally blind children being identified before the age of 2 years. Before routine surveillance only one-half had come to light by this age. This indicates that a system can greatly improve identification and that without it even serious handicaps can be neglected and remain undetected.

In one general practice, screening procedures led to the identification and referral of 30 children aged under 5 years for ophthalmic opinion – the highest number to any one specialty[11].

Therefore, some sort of screening programme which will not miss serious defects of acuity or alignment and which will not throw up false-positives in any quantity must be constructed. This programme must naturally take local conditions of professional expertise and premises into account.

The scheme presented here (see Table 2) attempts to make screening selective. This is realistic because of the shortage of professionals willing to undertake the work and also because the normal is the rule and the time taken to prove it universally is unprofitable. Screening is regarded as unnecessary by many parents, becoming even more suspect if doubts are raised about visual capacity in a particular child, causing unconfirmed anxiety. Therefore the groups selected for screening should be indicated by a clear rationale which parents are likely to accept.

The re-examination times in this plan are flexible to some extent. In certain young children where poor rapport seems to have a major influence on the results or whose concentration is fleeting, two or three tests at (say) monthly intervals may be necessary to establish consistent results. When in doubt the better acuity should be provisionally accepted, as very young children cannot achieve an acuity which is false (if the test is properly administered), but they may fall short for all sorts of reasons unrelated to their vision (but see myopia, p. 63).

In principle, clinics outside hospital staffed or advised by hospital ophthalmologists are to be preferred to hospital clinics, though geography and availability must play a considerable part in the decision. Children fare better at children's clinics than in mixed-age clinics, which are customary in most hospitals.

Defaulters are fewer in GP and community clinics and are better handled in these local clinics rather than in hospitals. Local children's eye clinics are accustomed to handling doubtful and unco-operative cases, which are often not so easily handled in busy hospital clinics.

Many local eye clinics have an orthoptist who has all the necessary skills for testing acuity as well as special techniques for diagnosing squints. These afford a good staging post, where the majority of doubtful or equivocal patients can be saved from going to hospital and where essential refraction can be performed. Continuity of staff with local knowledge is important and these clinics can provide it. Few, if any, have opticians on the staff, but their help would be highly valuable.

The screening programme requires some expertise and the GP or community physician undertaking the work would be helped by an intensive short course of training, though a great deal can be achieved with very little.

ACUITY TESTING AND DIFFICULTIES

Older children often underperform and need to be encouraged to read more lines than they wish to. When they come to a halt a line or two more is often achieved if they are asked to guess. On the other hand, the older myope soon becomes adept at momentarily peering through his lids, which greatly improves his acuity. This trick needs to be detected by careful observation.

Although the acuity without glasses is important, it is generally more important to know what it is with glasses. Both should be entered in the case notes. The acuity with glasses is the critical one in those who are going to become permanent wearers of glasses – even if only part-time.

A major source of error in testing is inefficient occlusion. A useful method is an adhesive patch of light strapping such as Dermocell which peels off the face cleanly and painlessly. Another effective occluder is the spring clip which is neat, comfortable and intriguing rather than frightening. A pinhole is an

Table 2 A screening schedule

Age	*Groups*	*Screen for*
Birth	All	Abnormalities of pupil funct Transparency of visual path Red reflex Gross structure Motility
By end of 1st year	Gross retardation Gross physical handicap Deaf	
	Constant squint Grossly abnormal visual behaviour	
	Inconstant squint	
By end of 2nd year	Constant squints Inconstant squints	
	Behaviour problems Suspected visual defect Retarded Physically handicapped	→ Binocular acuity
By end of 3rd year	Siblings of known squints Family history of early onset of visual defect Deaf	→ Acuity in each eye
	Defaulters and omissions Twins	→ Acuity in each eye
By school entry	All	Near and distance acuity
	Boys	Colour vision
Aged 7, 9, 11 and 13	All	Distance acuity
Older children		On demand only

Findings	*Disposal*
Obvious and constant abnormality	Ophthalmologist
Doubtful and inconstant abnormality	Re-examine in a month
	Paediatric assessment centres (combined with ophthalmologist)
	Ophthalmologist
	Keep under observation
	Ophthalmologist
Good	No action
Equivocal	Retest in 3 months
Defective	Ophthalmologist
Good acuity	No action
Equivocal Defective	Children's eye clinic for refraction and orthoptist
Good	No action
Gross defects (6/18 or worse) Unequal acuity (more than one line)	Clinic for refraction
Equivocal Minor defects (6/12 or better and equal)	Repeat and observe
6/9 distance in each 6/6 = near	Retest in 1 year
6/12 distance; 6/9 = near or worse	Refraction
Equivocal	Retest in 1 year
Defective	Inform parents and teachers
Defect previously recognized and stationary	No action
Progressive defects corrected by glasses to 6/9 or better	Check every 6 months
New defects Progressive defects not corrected by glasses to 6/9 or better	refraction

accepted device to indicate the level acuity may reach when glasses are ordered so it is obvious that occlusion must be complete or it will produce a pinhole effect and a false acuity in children with refractive anomalies. It is sometimes possible (notably in squinting children) to guess ahead which eye is likely to perform badly. It is wise to test this eye first, especially at re-examination, which prevents those with good memories seeming to produce better vision in one eye than is actually present. It is also good practice to obscure the test type before it is used or to divert the older child's attention somehow during the preliminaries. A useful form of occlusion in children who wear glasses is to lay a face tissue between the glasses and the eye. These are easily available, familiar and comfortable in addition to being totally effective if properly placed.

Myopia is usually progressive, sometimes 1 D or more in 6 months, though this rate is usually found only in younger myopes (say 6–10 years). For this reason amongst others a deterioration of even more than one line in older children must indicate a need to shorten the intervals between tests and to remember that even in known myopes the cause may be pathological. This can be excluded if acuity through a pinhole is 6/6, and there are no other abnormalities noted.

To save time and encourage concentration it is useful to place a coloured strip between the lines for 6/18 and 6/12 so that the child can be asked to start below it half-way down the chart (Figure 19: facing p. 65). Young children (say under 10) often misunderstand this instruction, but in older children screening time can be halved. Another method of saving time in younger literate children is to use a single-letter test type as in Figure 20 but care must be taken to ensure that memory does not affect the exercise.

In older children amblyopia in one eye which has been previously recognized and investigated requires no special attention, but routine testing of the good eye must not be neglected. Good documentation of all tests will relieve patients and the clinic staff of needless investigation of an old stable defect for which there is no effective treatment or relief after (say) 8 years old.

As far as possible, a distance of 6 m (20 ft) between patient and test type must be strictly adhered to and any variation mentioned. Illumination should be standard (therefore

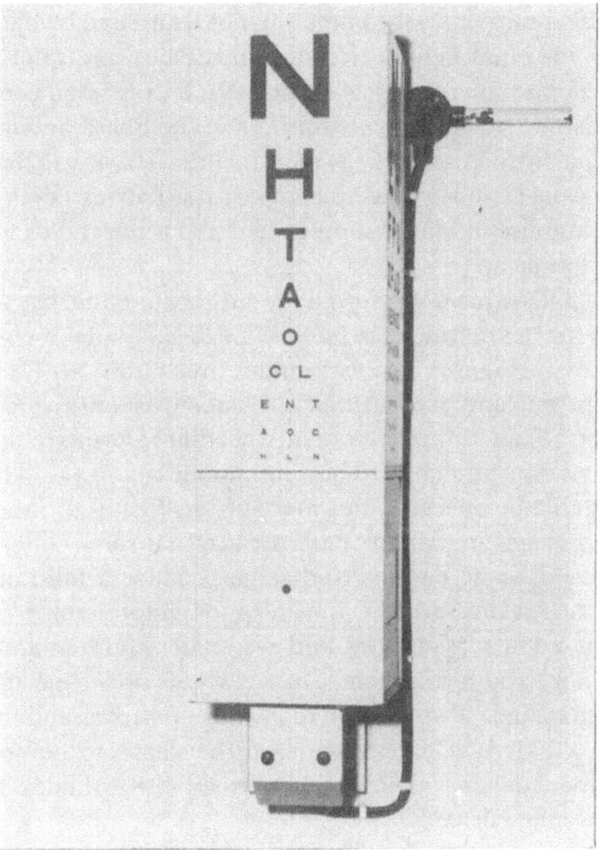

Figure 20 Single letter test type

artificial) and no shadows, streaks or rays should fall across the test chart or across the patient's face. The next best arrangement is a distance of 3 m (10 ft) into a mirror with the chart hung above the patient's head. This has the added advantage of enabling the examiner to point to letters he wants read out to him without a 12-metre walk, but some younger children (those under 5) are more confused by a mirror than by the direct method. They may fail to concentrate from such a distance so the use of a 3-metre (10 ft) distance chart may be forced. This must be indicated in the notes and not translated by halving to obtain the equivalent, as for clinical reasons this is not always correct. Also, there are few charts with letters small enough to establish a 6/6 equivalent from 3 m. The Sheridan Gardiner material (orthoptic version) does include 6/3 print. However, in the range 6/60–6/9 valid comparisons between eyes can be made and useful information gained about the child's possible visual handicap.

The apparatus necessary in the surgery or clinic has already been referred to, but no reference has been made to screening machines (Figure 21). Screening machines are carefully thought out and are sensitive, perhaps oversensitive in some respects. They do away with the need for a 6-metre distance between type and child. They are mobile but heavy. They are boring for the operator, but more or less foolproof. The great disadvantages in younger children are that some children are frightened, some dazzled and some produce a false myopia. Thus the use of a screening machine for children under the age of 10 is not a total success and even older children are sometimes not happy with them. On the whole, under the age of 10 these machines throw up too many false-positives and they are better avoided. If for convenience they have to be used the presumed defect should be confirmed by orthodox testing before being referred.

Hysterical or functional defective vision occurs occasionally. This is characteristically in girls, seldom complete but bad enough to be incapacitating. It is therefore usually exhibited as reduced vision in both eyes, though sometimes in one eye only. It seldom occurs before the age of 10 and is commonest between this age and 16. Inconsistency of performance is not necessarily

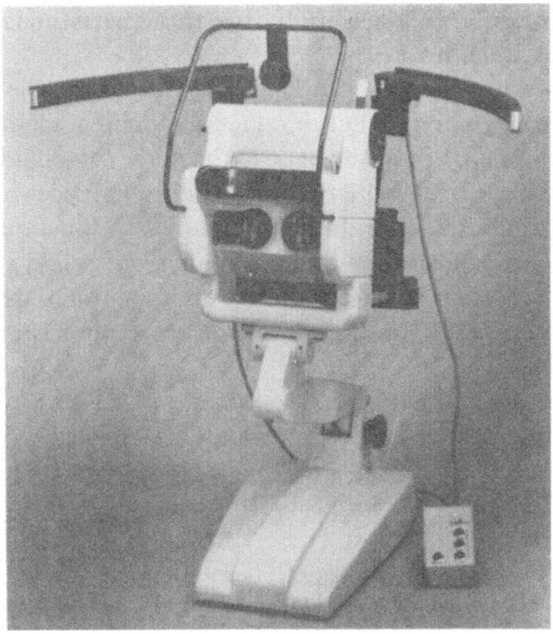

Figure 21 Keystone Vision Screener with electronic perimeter [by kind permission of C. Davis Keeler Ltd.]

a feature, but there is quite often incompatibility between near and distance performance, one or the other being more seriously affected than would be expected. Some will watch television but cannot see the blackboard. A suspicion should arise if a sudden onset is claimed, i.e. in a matter of days or hours, especially if it is bilateral; careful history taking is rewarding. Some will give up reading but continue to sew or to feed themselves without eating small fish bones. The varieties are endless. Proof in the consulting room is difficult without lenses or a prism bar. The prism bar will show a deviation which cannot occur in a blind eye, though it could in a defective eye. The most reliable method of detection is by use of dummy or neutralized lenses. The child will see more the more lenses that are piled on. Four lenses may be arranged and as each one is added the child will see a line or two more, even though the net power of the lenses is nil.

Recovery is the rule but it is worth exploring the cause to reassure the parent. The commonest cause is some tension or clash in school, but this may be in the home. Alcoholic fathers, criminal fathers and premature sexual experiences have been known as causes. It is unsafe to diagnose a functional defect without a demonstration that the vision is not as bad as it seems and it is wise to review after an interval if symptoms persist, but only if they do so. Constant reviewing leads to persistence of the condition.

There are several other tricks which will diagnose functional defects but these usually require ophthalmological ingenuity.

COLOUR VISION

There is no evidence that defects in colour vision vary in prevalence as a developmental process, though in very early childhood it is difficult to judge the sensory response to colour stimuli accurately.

Colour values alter in good illumination compared with poor. This is because the rods are responsible for twilight and night vision and response to colour is a cone function. Many pathological processes in the retina lead to modified colour response, but these are not a normal concern of developmental medicine.

It is a mistake to talk of 'colour blindness'. This is extremely rare and can be disregarded. However, defective colour vision is common in boys, roughly 8%, and one-tenth as common in girls. It is a sex-linked inherited defect and probably has a variable prevalence in different races.

Children begin to name colours accurately at about 3 years, though others take longer. This has little to do with their colour appreciation and is a reflection of their literacy more than of their vision, just as naming letters is.

Those that have a defect are likely to be unaware of the

reason why they make mistakes and so are their parents. This is not as strange as it sounds and arises from adaptation. For example, grass is always green (or brown) and the child will know that it must be inaccurate to call it red. He also knows that the colours of traffic lights are one of three appearing in different positions and orderly sequences. In addition each colour has a different luminosity so that identification can be made much more accurately than one would expect. Pillar boxes are always red, which eliminates naming the colour wrongly and so on. Yet in certain lights and possibly in certain environments the child might not recognize the pillar box as early in development as a normal child, nor as quickly against a confusing background.

The difficulties arise in trick positions, e.g. sorting out coloured marbles and judging the ripeness of tomatoes – and however accurate a child may be with traffic signals the clues he uses are gone if he takes to the water and has to judge masthead lights or the colours of buoys. The adaptation is believed to be so good that some of these boys go to art school and only then does it become apparent that there is a colour problem, leading (it is said) to a drift to pottery or sculpture rather than painting. Medical students with such a defect have some difficulty in interpreting microscope slides, and chemical titrations and such exercises can be a problem. As with so many defects the individual learns as a child to adapt and to dodge situations where he suspects there will be some difficulty. What he is reluctant to do is to report the difficulty and later to disclose it, except when he is forced to.

There is some evidence that the period of greatest difficulty is in the early years at school. This may be difficult to identify and the child may be held up to ridicule in class for making absurd mistakes for which he can himself see no reason. Though most teaching methods using colour differentials are based on a knowledge of the difficulty, it is a marginal disadvantage to have this clue in teaching blurred rather than clear. Those that are distressed are not likely to be cheered by the knowledge that owing to their defect they can see through certain types of camouflage and therefore in wartime have their special niche.

Since colour vision does not change in childhood or later, except from pathological causes, and because of the chances of difficulties arising at school, it seems sensible to test boys for colour vision problems at school entry. Speed and simplicity are the basic requirements in tests at this age and if versatility can be added to this so that the handicapped can be tested also it is an advantage. There are no tests that are completely reliable at this age, but a matching test similar to the Sheridan–Gardiner black and white test is available, known as the Guy's Colour Vision Test (see p. 56). Though it throws up a number of equivocal results the truly red/green defective are easily identified and it is only these who are likely to run into trouble. The Ishihara test depends on naming rather than matching and on tracing, both of which are difficult to interpret in young children, but has stood the test of time for older children. Other tests come and go and all have their recommendation.

In practice it is best to inform the teacher as well as the parent when a well-marked defect is found and to keep quiet about doubtful performers, suggesting a retest after 2 or 3 years.

The dividend in testing girls is so small that it is probably only worth testing those who come from families where colour vision is known to be defective.

GENETIC AND VISUAL HANDICAP OF EARLY ONSET[12]

Some of the commoner pathological conditions and syndromes with visual and genetic components early in life are listed below, but this is by no means extensive[13]. Textbooks on ophthalmology or paediatrics should be consulted on this topic.

(1) Buphthalmos.
(2) Albinism.

(3) Galactosaemia.
(4) Tay-Sachs disease.
(5) Amblyopia.
(6) Defective colour vision.
(7) Marfan's syndrome (subluxation of the lens).
(8) Sickle-cell anaemia.
(9) Stargardt's disease (muscular dystrophy).
(10) Leber's disease.
(11) Cataract.
(12) Nystagmus.
(13) Colobomata.
(14) Squint.
(15) Corneal dystrophy.
(16) Diabetes.
(17) Lowe's syndrome.
(18) Sturge–Weber syndrome.
(19) Down's syndrome.
(20) Tapeto-retinal degenerations.
(21) Rubella syndrome.

Generally, few children with serious visual defects of genetic origin are likely to appear in any one area and handling these therefore becomes a specialized activity. Their visual problems are mostly no different in effect from those of other children, though their potential for improvement is obviously less. Normally those conditions which arise early in life are adapted to and the best is made of limited vision.

Progressive conditions such as retinitis pigmentosa produce more problems because the age of manifestation is variable and so is the rate of deterioration. Incapacity may not arise until well into adult life in some and in others special schooling becomes necessary from an early age. These differences arise even within a family, which causes anxiety and confusion in the parents' minds.

Electropotential measurements are useful, though translating these into practical estimates or prognoses on which a programme can be based is still difficult[14]. In common with all adults the blind or partially sighted parent will judge their child's situation on the basis of their own experience. This is unlikely to be strictly parallel to the child's visual capacity; but doctors and some teachers, on the other hand, tend to put too much stress on the actual figures they are given. 6/60 vision may seem to many to indicate incapacity, yet the parent may have been carrying out all essential activities without great difficulty with this degree of acuity. Attempts to categorize patients as partially sighted or blind, particularly children, are bound to have big margins of error because what use the child will make of his limited vision is unknown and until this is settled the degree of handicap is also unknown. The loss of both legs might be reasonably supposed to put an end to playing golf, yet individuals have gone back to the game.

REGISTRATION PROCEDURE

Registration as blind or partially sighted is not statutory but voluntary. Hence the discrepancies found when thorough local surveys are performed. There are always more people with visual defects which would qualify than the official statistics show – particularly the partially sighted. This also partly accounts for very large differences in statistics from one area to another. Registration opens the door to aids and benefits – whether of training, finance, appliances etc. – but oddly it is not required by all authorities for special education. Apart from this there are large numbers of blind or partially sighted children in mental health institutions who are not registered, either because they have not been recognized as such or because no benefits would follow.

The registration document (the B.D.8) has to be signed by a consultant ophthalmologist. This is a safeguard against errors made by well-meaning practitioners who may not be aware of the difficulties of diagnosis and prognosis. I have seen children in special schools who have never been examined by a consultant ophthalmologist, and who have been wrongly diagnosed as partially sighted, though not registered, and accepted as such by the school health authorities. I have also seen paramedical practitioners attempting futile and demanding exercises from blind patients, assuming that they could see because they were not registered.

Registration is, however, a cumbersome procedure and very demoralizing for parents or older children with its label and seeming quality of irrevocability. For educational purposes not only is it not always required, but final decisions about places and methods of education are in the hands of the education authorities, who may well be guided by the S.E.2 certificate, the ophthalmic content of which is inadequately formulated and often also incompletely written.

The B.D.8 is held by the social services department, who should be approached by anybody (medical or otherwise) who believes that a person may be severely visually handicapped. The individual's particular circumstances determine what should be the next move, but the most direct procedure is to go straight for a consultant's opinion, bearing in mind that he will need medical details before signing the document. There are often difficulties of disposal in cases of multiple handicap which are best dealt with by paediatric assessment teams – whether formal or informal. There are also several children, particularly infants, whose vision is impossible to assess within the accuracies required and with any degree of finality. These children require frequent review and several who give no visual response in infancy are examples of delayed visual maturation. Eventually they turn out to have useful or even normal vision[15 16].

These children particularly (and their advisers) require more ophthalmic help than is always provided either at developmental clinics or in the early years at school. The educationally subnormal present particular problems of cause and effect which are not easily assessed in a routine hospital outpatient ophthalmic clinic.

The term 'residual vision' is in common use amongst those who work with the visually handicapped; it means vision which cannot accurately be measured. Usually it is worse than 1/60 and includes field defects of all kinds.

Those who seem to have intact peripheral visual apparatus but no vision are stated to be cortically blind. Apart from some traumatic cases and those with cerebral tumours, all of these children are retarded or brain damaged from birth and suffer from microcephaly.

Many of the conditions with a familial factor are in a sense trivial, but a higher proportion of the blind and partially sighted come from families which know something about the disease from first-hand experience. The task of the doctor is to exercise special vigilance in screening such families and to see that special educational assessments are made promptly, as well as accepting some responsibility for mobilizing the social services immediately a handicap develops.

The special problems of the visually handicapped child are very unevenly met in different areas of the country and are seldom totally dealt with. One of the difficulties is relating ophthalmic reports written in professional jargon to the visual performance of the child. Even the comparatively direct terms 'blind' and 'partially sighted' do not mean what they seem to mean, though they have statutory definitions. Only about 5% of those correctly registered as blind have no vision – many function very well in familiar surroundings, especially if the defect begins early in life. The most severely handicapped amongst the partially sighted are those who cannot read, but this is not part of the statutory definition. No wonder the doctor is initially confused.

However, a commonsense assessment regardless of statutes or labels can be made of a specific child's needs provided that the information about his vision is accurate and comprehensible. There is one small group which demands special attention and is not easily identified. This is the group whose vision fluctuates. Generally, the acuity of partially sighted schoolchildren is likely to be stable. Some improve, more with learning than organically; but certain diseases (Still's disease being one), some dystrophies, some therapies, etc. may provide periods of excellent vision for weeks and months, intermittent with bouts of poor vision. These are quite unforeseeable and of uncertain eventual prognosis. There are also children who are apt to suffer deterioration, notably hydrocephalics, where this may be the first signal of serious intracranial complications.

The teacher's report, if possible by word of mouth, is desirable in giving educational advice. Difficulties often arise because the teacher is confused and may even be afraid of damaging the child's eyes and refrains from demanding visual tasks over which the child is in difficulty. This may lead to asking too little of the child or unwittingly too much.

The school doctor needs to have some system in conjunction with the teachers and ophthalmologist so that handicapped children with visual difficulties are under frequent review. The community or school medical and ophthalmic services should be easily accessible and unrestricted by too much protocol. The parent must be informed when a defect is first discovered or has changed, but most need to be helped to get the right advice. This is not necessarily a one-off visit to hospital, where the child will be seen by a stranger who may only have a rather garbled story from the parent. Such children need to present (but not at the cost of too much time) a proper account of the circumstances in school or in general development which have precipitated the referral.

Services may well be provided by a paediatric assessment centre with on-call ophthalmic help. The handicapped child in a normal school is rather more at risk of not having confident teachers who understand the issues, nor do they have a visiting ophthalmologist who can give first-hand advice on the individual problems in the particular setting. Schools for the handicapped, whatever other contentions there may be about their value, are usually much better placed for adequate medical and ophthalmic supervision – or ought to be.

The ideal provision of services is difficult to achieve, because the numbers and distribution of children with these handicaps are small and widely spread out. Schools for the blind, therefore, mainly have to be boarding schools; and schools for the partially sighted are often too far for daily attendance. This difficulty leads inevitably to some of these children being placed in normal school, where it is hoped that proper help is available.

Another disadvantage of normal school is the psychological drawback of being conspicuous. An albino will be most unlikely to find another like himself except at a special school. This also applies to children with nystagmus. These children are conspicuous not only because of their peculiar eye movements but also because they need to hold reading matter about $2\frac{1}{2}$ cm (1 in) from their eyes (Figure 22). Their performance at this distance may be normal. Similarly, children who use magnifiers or watchmaker's glasses to read are at a psychological disadvantage in normal school. This is understandable when compared with the normal child's abhorrence of glasses because they make him feel overexposed.

VISUAL AIDS

These include all forms of telescopes and magnifiers. It is tempting to overrate the benefit from the use of aids. Reading large print without an aid is easier than reading small print with a magnifier. This is because all magnifiers and telescopes restrict the field of vision and scanning is not possible. Once a child has learnt to read, however, he becomes surprisingly nimble with a magnifier, whether hand-held (Figure 23(a)) or in spectacle frames (Figure 23(b)), provided he is keen and interested. Similarly, in the distance a panoramic view is difficult to achieve with a visual aid, especially if the user is in motion. However, some children's exploratory efforts with a telescopic device are encouraged if, for instance, they can see a street name or a station indicator board.

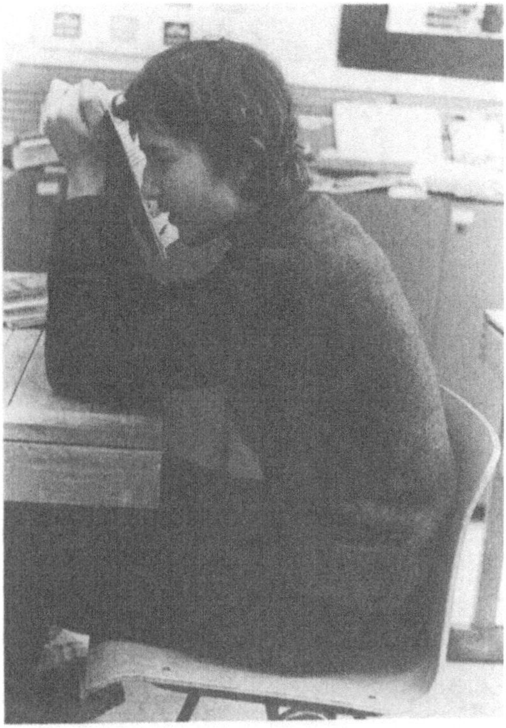

Figure 22 A visually handicapped reader (John Aird School) [© Peter Fowler]

Generally speaking, aids are not used willingly by children aged under 10, and those older than this who are likely to use them are best quietly introduced to the idea and their reaction studied during an arranged trial period. There will be considerable waste if aids are issued on a rule of thumb basis to all whose acuity is improved.

Use of an aid is accepted in special schools by the wearer much more readily than in a normal school. This does not apply to closed-circuit television, but for an individual the expense is a deterrent. Closed circuit television is a boon to the visually handicapped. Figures 24 and 25 show how normal

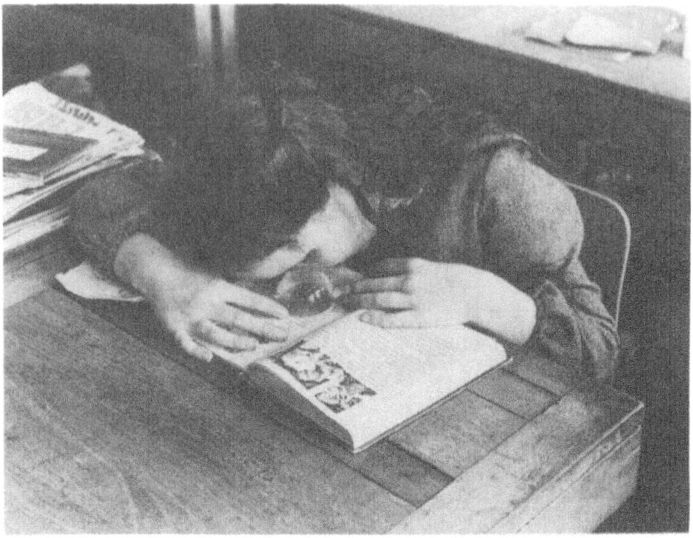

(a)

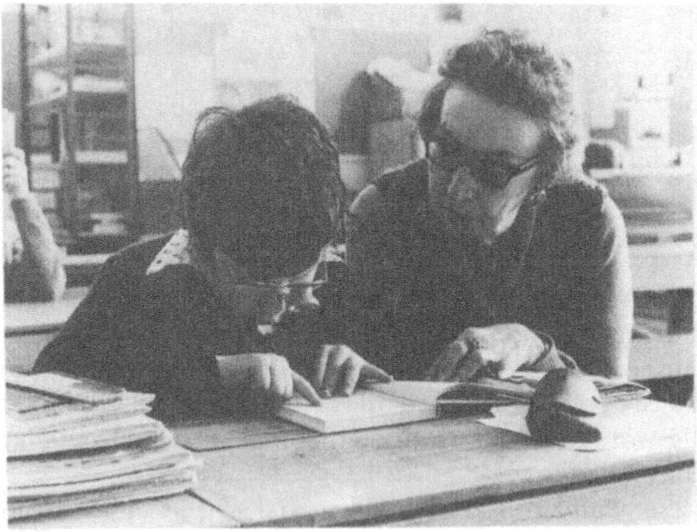

(b)

Figure 23(a) and (b) Useful magnifiers for the visually handicapped (John Aird School) [© Peter Fowler]

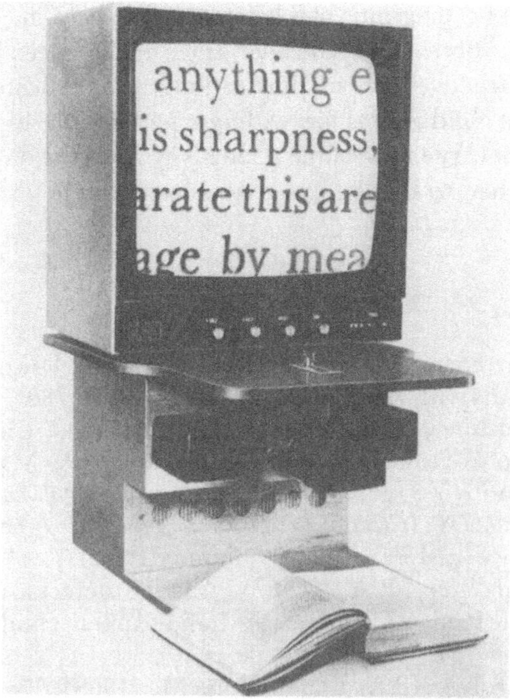

Figure 24 Closed-circuit television – enlargement of reading print

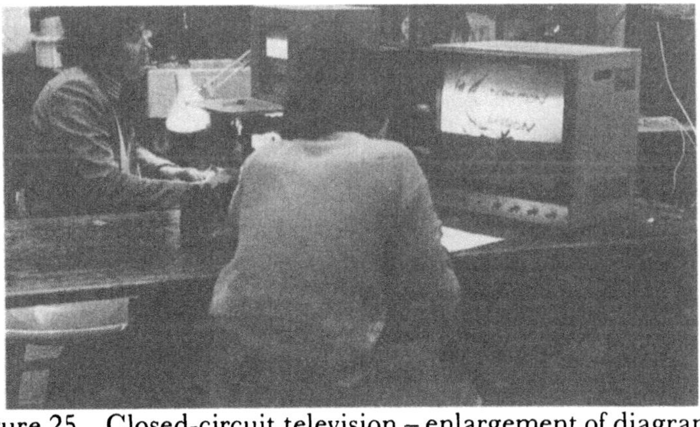

Figure 25 Closed-circuit television – enlargement of diagram [© Peter Fowler]

reading and diagrams can be enlarged to help in reading and teaching. Both these considerations make special schooling more attractive. These illustrations also indicate that any posture a child adopts for reading is permissible, especially if it is essential. We have come a long way from the days when all reading had to be performed at a 'respectable' distance from the print.

References

1. Gardiner, P.A. and Peckham, C. (1980). Use of glasses by adolescents with good vision. *Br. Med. J.*, **281**, 780

2. Gardiner, P.A. (1969). The 'At risk' concept with reference to visual disorders. In Gardiner, P., MacKeith, R. and Smith, V. (eds.) *Aspects of Developmental and Paediatric Ophthalmology* (*Clinics in Developmental Medicine* No. 32) (London: S.I.M.P. with Heinemann Medical)

3. Gardiner, P.A. (1967). Visual defects in Down's syndrome and other mentally handicapped children. *Br. J. Ophthalmol.*, **51**, 7

4. Gardiner, P.A. and Joseph, M. (1968). Eye defects in children with congenital heart lesions: a preliminary study. *Dev. Med. Child Neurol.*, **10** (1)

5. Gardiner, P.A. (1969). Refractive errors in relation to physical characteristics and systemic disorders. In Gardiner, P., MacKeith, R. and Smith, V. (eds.) *Aspects of Developmental and Paediatric Ophthalmology* (*Clinics in Developmental Medicine* No. 32) (London: S.I.M.P. with Heinemann Medical)

6. Black, P.D. (1980). Ocular defects in children with cerebral palsy. *Br. Med. J.*, **281**, 487–488

7. Raikes, A. (1979). Preliminary visual screening. In Smith, V. and Keen, J. (eds.) *Visual Handicap in Children* (*Clinics in Developmental Medicine* No. 73) (London: S.I.M.P. with Heinemann Medical)

8. Smith, V.H. (1979). The Birmingham Orthoptic Screening Service. In Smith, V. and Keen, J. (eds.) *Visual Handicap in Children* (*Clinics in Developmental Medicine* No. 73) (London: S.I.M.P. with Heinemann Medical)

9. Gardiner, P.A. (1974). Squint diagnostic clinics. *Trans. Ophthalmol. Soc. UK*, **94** (1)

10. Jan, J., Freeman, R.D. and Scott, E.P. (1977). *Visual Impairment in Children and Adolescents* (New York: Grune and Stratton)

11. Jenkins, G.H.C., Collins, C. and Andrew, S. (1978). Developmental surveillance in general practice. *Br. Med. J.*, **1**, 1537–1540

12. Jay, B. (1979). Genetic causes of visual handicap: prevalence and prevention. In Smith, V. and Keen, J. (eds.) *Visual Handicap in Children* (*Clinics in Developmental Medicine* No. 73) (London: S.I.M.P. with Heinemann Medical)

13. Mellor, D. (1979). Hereditary syndromes associated with neurological disorder and early visual handicap. In Smith, V. and Keen, J. (eds.) *Visual Handicap in Children* (*Clinics in Developmental Medicine* No. 73) (London: S.I.M.P. with Heinemann Medical)

14. Galloway, N.R. (1979). The value of electro-diagnostic tests in the diagnosis of inherited retinal degenerations. In Smith, V. and Keen, J. (eds.) *Visual Handicap in Children* (*Clinics in Developmental Medicine* No. 73) (London: S.I.M.P. with Heinemann Medical)

15. Illingworth, R.S. (1961). Delayed visual maturation. *Arch. Dis. Child.*, **36**, 407

16. Rosenbloom, L. (1979). The phenomenon of delayed visual maturation. *Neuropadiatrie*, **Suppl. 10**, 447 (abstract)

Chapter 7

VISUAL DEVELOPMENT IN THE HANDICAPPED CHILD

Visual defects of all sorts are more common in children suffering from other handicaps from birth or early childhood than amongst normal children. These defects are in addition to those which are part of recognized syndromes of abnormality. Therefore, special attention should be given to identifying the visual handicap of these children with a view to improving their lot socially and educationally and determining those (the minority) who might be helped by medical measures; easing the burden of those who care for them is part of this. The difficulties of examining these children and of coming to a definitive statement on acuity are very much greater than in normal children, though in practice the clinical questions to be answered for brain-damaged and retarded children of any age are similar to those for normal infants.

Special difficulties show themselves in different ways and have a special importance:

(1) Does the visual difficulty, if any, play any part in the child's retardation, whether physical or mental?
(2) How much treatment (such as a normal child might receive in a given condition) will be justified in a child with other abnormalities (e.g. a child with rubella syndrome, squint and refractive error)?
(3) How should some sort of special service for special

problems be organized in view of the difficulties of getting children like this to hospital? (This may be determined by going to schools and centres.)

It is quite common in normal young children to find that their personality alters if they are given glasses which overcome a visual defect. Commonly this manifests itself as their becoming less shy and more adventurous, sometimes within a matter of days and as young as 2 years old. In school attainment standards of work can improve dramatically. It would be pleasant to record that this type of behaviour modification can be produced in the retarded, but it is very uncommon. A high-grade mongol girl aged 7 years was regarded as exceptionally affectionate and well motivated because of her taking her teacher's hand out of class and always coming up to table in class to participate in what was being demonstrated. When she was found (by chance) to be highly myopic and was given glasses these traits disappeared. This is a classical example of misjudgement by adults of the real foundation of a behaviour and personality pattern. This misjudgement was accepted by her doctors without question. Although there was a modification of behaviour, its nature and timing was unexpected.

A major difficulty in the way of improving acuity in retarded children is obtaining their consent to wearing glasses. Their refusal is often reasonable. In the first place they become a target for their schoolmates, as many a normal child has found but can overcome. It is more difficult to discipline the retarded. Secondly, in younger children one often can only assume that the glasses are beneficial since tests of acuity are so often equivocal. As the child matures it may become apparent that the glasses are not providing a major benefit, if any. This can even happen with children who started wearing glasses at a young age and are upset if they are without them.

As for glasses, very young retarded children can sometimes be persuaded to wear them (though not so often to care for them) much as they wear clothes. This attitude can be extended to their demanding to wear them later in childhood or being distressed if they are lost. This may occur even if the glasses are proved to have little influence on their vision.

These factors are apt to be understood with difficulty by the hospital consultant unless he has comprehensive reports from all those in daily contact with the child.

A notable example of this was an aphakic boy who after having his cataracts removed in infancy was given +10.0 D lenses which he wore initially with persuasion but later at his own insistence. An accidental trial of −10 D lenses showed that he was happier with these than without any glasses, proving that he was accustomed to having glasses of any strength on his nose and that what he saw through them was irrelevant.

At the other end of the scale a mongol who was capable of matching tests was found to have a distance acuity of 6/60 with each eye and when provided with glasses an acuity of 6/9 in each eye. He was re-examined after 12 months and to everyone's satisfaction, including his own, showed no change in this acuity. However, it was noticed that as soon as he left the examination room he took off the spectacles, placed them with great care in their case and put the case in his jacket. Enquiry showed that he seldom wore his glasses, reserving them for full-dress occasions, but that they were one of his most treasured possessions.

Therefore in severely retarded children of any age, it is often impossible to determine before a trial with glasses is conducted, whether the visual defect plays any part in the child's general progress. This is partly because it is unknown how much acuity will improve with glasses and partly because there is doubt in those children whose acuity does improve whether it may not be intolerable. This is not as odd as it might seem. Many normal myopes take off their glasses to give their eyes a rest and every ophthalmologist knows that to give anyone 6/5 vision or better, regardless of their previous acuity, is risky because there will often be complaints that the world is too clear. This is analogous to difficulties arising in the deaf when an aid is worn.

The amount of information fed in is overwhelming. To a lesser extent this applies to the educationally subnormal also.

The best practice seems to be to refract all the retarded and to order a trial of glasses where major anomalies are found, usually for constant wear. In this case they will not be lost or broken as often as when they are worn only part-time. If glasses are started in infancy they may become part of a child's clothing and accepted as such. This at least gives a child the opportunity of seeing well. As with any young child consistent refusal may indicate that acuity is worse with glasses than without and it must be remembered that it takes time for full acuity with glasses to come about in young children, particularly if they are high hypermetropes or astigmats. This difference from myopes may be because myopes have clear near vision to build on, however bad their distance vision. This process of development may be even more prolonged or absent in the retarded.

When glasses have been consistently refused or worn for only short periods it is probably wise to give up their use altogether unless there is very strong positive evidence that they are of visual benefit. Under the age of 10 it is always worth trying again after an interval.

SQUINTS IN THE HANDICAPPED

The general rationale of treating squints is recorded elsewhere (see p. 88). The special considerations relating to the retarded and handicapped are:

(1) The goal of full binocular vision is even less likely to be reached in either than it is in normal children.
(2) Treatment with occlusion is even more onerous than it is for normal children.
(3) Surgery for only cosmetic reasons is less desirable.
(4) There is increased risk to the child's general health whether from brain damage, anoxia, chest or cardiac

disease, particularly in those with congenitally defective hearts or lungs or diminished resistance to infection.
(5) The risk that some general gain such as walking or talking already acquired late may be affected detrimentally. Enthusiasm for treatment of the eyes in these children must be balanced against the possible harm to general development.

These children, particularly the brain damaged, have a considerably higher rate of prevalence of squint and the squints appearing are often of bizarre types with more than the average number of vertical and divergent squints amongst them. Their acuity is more difficult to assess, their reaction to anaesthetics may be alarming and they can be less co-operative than normal children. Their mothers, with some justification, become impatient about numerous lengthy journeys and protracted periods of treatment. This must not lead to doing nothing at all and investigation is as necessary as in normal children, but treatment must be considered more in the light of what might easily and quickly benefit that particular child rather than aim at eventual perfection. These children tolerate glasses badly (with notable exceptions) and can become generally disturbed during occlusion, reverting to more infantile behaviour patterns such as bed wetting.

It is usually wiser to settle for a good cosmetic result in those who are likely to be out in the world and even to abandon this for those (the most mentally retarded) who are unlikely to be seriously disadvantaged by their appearance. These children are, of course, mostly in institutions or are too retarded to mix with those outside the home. None of this absolves the doctor from full initial investigation and review at regular intervals.

One guide is the likely gain in overall acuity against the visual handicap present and its effects. Clearly, blindness will demand more active treatment, where possible, than a minor handicap, even against the odds of success. Since this occurs as a pathological condition and is not strictly a typical developmental problem except within its own characteristics, it is outside the scope of this book. Most squints occur in children with good vision and at worst adequate vision in one eye even if glasses are needed to achieve it. The visual problem therefore may become one of how far to pursue treatment to improve vision in an amblyopic eye.

Many would advise treatment only as long as it is no significant burden to parent or child. The burden of treatment can be heavy in retarded children or in those with considerable physical handicap.

SERVICES FOR HANDICAPPED CHILDREN

The principles on which services to the handicapped should be based are common to those for normal children – namely, early and comprehensive detection of visual defect and easily approached clinics where competent practitioners can decide whether ocular pathology is present, where refraction can take place and where follow-up can be organized. The General Ophthalmic Service is even less suitable for them than it is for normal children and their problems will not be understood.

There is a much higher incidence of visual defect in the retarded and the physically handicapped than in the normal population[1], but considerably more difficulty in organizing effective screening cover and follow-up. This arises largely from poor mobility and even if these children do come to clinics it is difficult to marry the management for normal children to the disruptive effects on timetables and behaviour problems which many of these children exhibit. This problem is even worse in normal mixed-age hospital outpatient departments.

A solution would be to provide special clinics or sessions for handicapped children only, supported by efficient transport. Even so, many of these children are disturbed by novel surroundings and a better alternative is to take the services to the children. This comprises periodic visits to institutions or schools by a peripatetic team which may consist of ophthalmologist, orthoptist, optician and paediatrician. The active co-operation of local health visitors, school nurses, social workers and the like is essential so that follow-on instructions can be given and explained to the child and his parents. Documentation must be strict and reports broadcast to all who deal with the child.

Paediatric assessment centres, whether community or hospital attached, should give special attention to the vision of the retarded and provide the necessary expertise without treading on each other's toes[2].

It is often believed that the equipment necessary for such a service is overwhelmingly expensive, but 90% of children can be adequately examined with a box of trial lenses, simple test types, portable orthoptic tests, an ophthalmoscope for fundus examination and a retinoscope for refraction, together with a diversity of cycloplegics. A van or caravan is desirable if the clinic itself has to be mobile in rural areas.

Successful pilot schemes have been run along these lines in rural and urban areas.

There remain the 10% or so who present diagnostic problems or where uncertainty arises out of difficulties with examination or who require active medical help. These need to be seen at hospital, but once the immediate difficulties are overcome they are likely to feel happier if they are referred back to local services, where these are well organized. These problems arise particularly in the younger child and it does not do to defer investigation until they are 'manageable'.

Too many retarded children have no informed opinion on them, are not looked at routinely and in many instances their vision is not taken into account by those who care for them. This is often because no report reaches those in daily contact with the child or if it does it is out of date or incomprehensible.

References

1. Tallents, C. (1979). The visual handicap found in a population of mentally and physically handicapped children. In

Smith, V. and Keen, J. (eds.) *Visual Handicap in Children* (*Clinics in Developmental Medicine* No. 73) (London: S.I.M.P. with Heinemann Medical)

2. Hunt, H., McKendrick, O., Poole, J., Pugh, R.E., Rosenbloom, L. and Turnock, R. (1979). Visual impairment in childhood. In Smith, V. and Keen, J. (eds.) *Visual Handicap in Children* (*Clinics in Developmental Medicine* No. 73) (London: S.I.M.P. with Heinemann Medical)

GLOSSARY

Accommodation Focusing the eye for near vision.

Acuity Measurement of visual function, commonly expressed as a fraction of what can be seen at 6 metres (20 ft); i.e. 6/60 (20/200) equals at 6 metres no better than a normal eye can see at 60 metres.

Amblyopia Defective acuity not compensated for by glasses and not accounted for by demonstrable pathology. A lazy eye.

Aniridia Absence of the iris.

Anisometropia As commonly used this is a marked difference in refraction between one eye and the other (say 2 dioptres or more whether spherical or astigmatic or both).

Buphthalmos Raised pressure in infantile eyes.

Ciliary muscle The muscle inside the globe responsible for focusing for near vision.

Cornea The transparent central front surface of the globe.

Cycloplegia Abolition of accommodation.

Dioptre	The numerical power of an optical system usually expressed as $\pm x$ D. Indicates the strength of spectacle lens.
Diplopia	Double vision.
Enophthalmos	A sunken eye.
Fixation	(normal) Looking directly at an object. (eccentric) Looking off target.
Fundus	The posterior segment of the interior of the globe.
General Ophthalmic Service	The normal free eye-testing carried out by opticians and some ophthalmologists.
Hypermetropia	Long sight, may cause difficulty with near vision.
Iris	The coloured tissue surrounding the pupil.
Macula	The area of the retina with the greatest concentration of cells responsive to light.
Medical eye centres	Consulting rooms attached to dispensing opticians' premises where an ophthalmological opinion can be obtained on the NHS. No introduction by the general practitioner is necessary, however desirable.
Miosis	Constriction of the pupil.
Mydriasis	Dilatation of the pupil.
Myelination	The process which completes the structure of nerve tissue.
Myopia	Short sight, always causes difficulty with distance vision.
Near vision	Material viewed from arm's length or less (conventionally 25 cm).

Occlusion	Covering an eye.
Ophthalmologist	A generic term for fully qualified doctors who later specialize in the diagnoses and treatment of visual defects and diseases.
Optician, dispensing	Professionals trained to fit and dispense spectacles from the prescriptions of ophthalmologists and, in some cases, of ophthalmic opticians (see medical eye centres).
Optician, ophthalmic	A non-medical practitioner concerned primarily with the detection of refractive anomalies and the provision of spectacles.
Optometrist	In the UK, synonymous with the above.
Orthoptics	That part of the supervision of squints and allied disorders other than surgical or optical.
Ptosis	Drooping of upper lid.
Refraction	The optical measurement of the eye.
Residual vision	Useful vision which is below the standardized measurements of acuity.
Retinoscopy	Measurement of refraction by light reflexes from the retina through the pupil.
Sclera	The white of the eye.
Snellen type	The standard chart used for sight testing.
Squint	Present when the two eyes are not looking at the same object.
Strabismus	Squint.
Visual cortex	The nerve cell layers in the brain which respond to visual input.

INDEX

GPSR Compliance

The European Union's (EU) General Product Safety Regulation (GPSR) is a set of rules that requires consumer products to be safe and our obligations to ensure this.

If you have any concerns about our products, you can contact us on ProductSafety@springernature.com

In case Publisher is established outside the EU, the EU authorized representative is:

Springer Nature Customer Service Center GmbH
Europaplatz 3
69115 Heidelberg, Germany

Batch number: 10584446

Printed by Printforce, the Netherlands